Leadership and Management in Healthcare

Stefan Abela

# Leadership and Management in Healthcare

## A Guide for Medical and Dental Practitioners

Springer

Stefan Abela
Oral Health Department
Norfolk and Norwich University Hospital NHS Foundation Trust
Norwich, UK

ISBN 978-3-031-21024-2 ISBN 978-3-031-21025-9 (eBook)
https://doi.org/10.1007/978-3-031-21025-9



This Springer imprint is published by the registered company Springer Nature Switzerland AG
The registered company address is: Gewerbestrasse 11, 6330 Cham, Switzerland

*This book is dedicated to my wife Dr. Milisha Chotai, my parents Joseph and Pauline Abela, my siblings Shawn and Maria Abela, sibling-in-law Charmaine and Andrew and my parents-in-law, Mrs. Sudha Chotai and in loving memory of Dr. Narendra Chotai.*

# Preface

Managing complex clinical scenarios is a part of everyday practice for hospital doctors, but these clinical management skills take time to acquire. Specialty training programmes in the UK are very thorough and train doctors to a very high clinical standard. However, training in hospital management is not part of the approved curriculum and in-depth guidance is often lacking or not provided at all. Final undergraduate students, trainees and newly appointed consultants, in particular, can be faced with complex management scenarios or may be tasked to solve crucial medical dilemmas. This is equally valid in real life on a daily basis or in very important interviews with little or no previous experience and knowledge on which to base their actions and responses.

A limited number of management skills can be acquired through specific training programmes, but experience can only be gained with time. There is no formal pathway to gain skills in this area and so this book aims to provide the information necessary to facilitate and increase the ability of trainees to address potential issues before they escalate.

Medical management and leadership is in a constant sphere of change. Changes are dictated by governmental administrators and providers alike with the ultimate aim being that of providing the ideal healthcare model. To this effect, some of the diagrams, management concepts and bodies could have been modified or replaced by the time this book is in full production.

This book provides general concepts and models and the reader should be aware of the subtle differences that can be found between the national health services in the different constituent countries that comprise the UK.

The author has, in the second part of the book attempted to outline strategies for dealing with the management problems that arise, often on a daily basis. The contents of this book will certainly increase the confidence of the reader preparing to face interviews, examinations and daily life as a medical or dental practitioner. It will also be invaluable in obtaining familiarity with the system if you are preparing to move oversees or if you are based in a commonwealth country with similar medical systems in place.

This book is ideal for final-year medical and dental undergraduate students, postgraduate students including foundation-year doctors, medical and dental core trainees, registrars, specialist practitioners and newly appointed consultants.

Norwich, UK
January 2023

Stefan Abela

# Junior and Academic Grades Nomenclature

| | |
|---|---|
| *Junior Medical Grades Positions* | |
| FY1 | Foundation year one junior doctor |
| FY2 | Foundation year two junior doctor |
| ST | Specialty trainee in a hospital specialty |
| SpR | Specialty registrar in a hospital specialty |
| GPST | Specialty registrar in general practice |
| *Junior Dental Grades Positions* | |
| DFT | Dental Foundation trainee (previously known as VT - Vocational training) |
| DCT1 | Dental Core Trainee year one dentist |
| DCT2 | Dental Core Trainee year two dentist |
| Dental StR | Dental Specialist trainee |
| Post-CCST | Post-Certificate of Completion of Specialist Training |
| *Academic Medical Grades Positions* | |
| ACF | Academic clinical fellow |
| CL | Clinical lecturer |
| CRF | Clinical research fellow |
| CSL | Senior clinical lecturer |
| RD | Reader |
| AP | Associate professor |
| Prof | Professor |

Definitions of harm from the National Reporting and Learning System (NRLS)

No harm:

- Impact prevented—any patient safety incident that had the potential to cause harm but was prevented, resulting in no harm to people receiving NHS-funded care.
- Impact not prevented—any patient safety incident that ran to completion, but no harm occurred to people receiving NHS-funded care.

Minor harm:

- Any patient safety incident that required extra observation, or minor treatment and caused minimal harm to one or more persons receiving NHS-funded care.

Moderate harm:

- Any patient safety incident that resulted in a moderate increase in treatment and which caused significant but not permanent harm, to one or more persons receiving NHS-funded care.

Major harm:

- Any patient safety incident that appears to have resulted in permanent harm to one or more persons receiving NHS-funded care.

Catastrophic harm (including death)

- Any patient safety incident that directly resulted in the death of one or more persons receiving NHS-funded care.

# Acknowledgements

I would like to thank the many people who saw me through the writing of this book and to all those who provided support, talked things over and encouraged me to persevere in seeing the book through to publication.

Heartfelt thanks go to my family, who supported and encouraged me. Above all, I would like to express my deepest gratitude to my wife, Dr. Milisha Chotai (DDS, PGCert, MSc, MSc), because her support and help never fail to surprise me. She has been invaluable and understanding in many ways, despite my commitment to the book taking me away from being close to her in times of need.

The final thanks should go to all those who have been involved in the peer-review process; William Mifsud, Harshini Pindolia, Nitin Thacker, Salehi Mahan, Ramayee Sivasubramanian, Issar Hussain , Catherine Liu, Ryan Seguna, Ajay Kumar, Ronnie Farrugia and John Cutajar amongst others and all those whose names I will not mention to ensure that nobody feels forgotten.

# Contents

# Part I

# The Management, Structure and Function of the National Health Service

# The Structure of the NHS 1

## 1.1 Introduction

The National Health Service (NHS) in England and Wales has gone through significant changes in both structure and funding streams in recent times. These changes were a result of The Health and Social Care Act (2012), with the legislative changes taking place in April 2013.

Historically, the NHS received all funds in annual lump sums known as 'block contracts'. This was a contractual agreement which meant that each hospital was entitled to receive the agreed funds, regardless of the level or quantity of service provided. In 2003, 'block contracts' were replaced by 'payment by results', which as the name suggests related payments to the amount of activity at each hospital. Today, the trend is to pay trusts based on the quality of care and health targets reached. The funding policy is usually set for a given period of time; however, an ongoing expectation of change is also very tangible. This flexibility allowed an emergency response fund in addition to a contingency fund announced by the government in response to the global COVID-19 pandemic.

In England and Wales, the total number of NHS trusts totals 217. An NHS trust refers to an organisational unit that provides healthcare within a specific geographical area and/or provides a very specialised type of care. A trust will therefore normally encompass multiple hospitals to provide the necessary coverage and ensure adequate public access.

There are 4 types of trusts:

- Acute health trusts.
- Ambulance trusts.
- Mental health trusts.
- Community health trusts.

 
S. Abela, *Leadership and Management in Healthcare*,
https://doi.org/10.1007/978-3-031-21025-9_1

NHS trusts were established under the National Health Service and Community Care Act 1990 and since then, several governmental directives have ensued to change their status to an NHS Foundation Trust. The latter nomenclature represents the legislative changes under the Community Health and Standards Act 2003 that entitles a trust to have greater financial autonomy and governance.

The various acute NHS Foundation trusts providing acute secondary care can be further classified into a University Teaching Hospitals (UTH) and District General Hospitals (DGH) with the former having a stronger research background, are affiliated to a medical university and have bigger departments with academic figureheads.

### 1.1.1 Funding Streams

The capital for NHS England has over the years consistently showed an upward trend possibly reflecting the nature of healthcare which is continuously advancing increasing the monetary demands on the healthcare budget provisions. The NHS England budget for 2018/2019 was set at £114.8 billion and rose to £133.4 billion in 2021/2022. The expected expenditure for 2023/2024 is set at £148.6 billion. 98.8% of the monies is provided from general taxation and National Insurance (NI) contributions whilst the remaining 1.2% is provided through patient charges.

This funding is subject to review every 2–3 years by Parliament unless the Chancellor of the Exchequer allocates additional funding by announcing it in the House of Commons at annual budget and gets the majority of the Parliament's approval. The majority of the funds are transferred to the Department of Health (DH) which then subsequently transfers it to NHS England, which funds all nationally commissioned services. NHS England is responsible for funding bodies such as Public Health England and the Clinical Commissioning Groups (CCGs) now defunct and replaced by Integrated Care Systems, ICSs. The latter is in turn responsible for commissioning services locally. Figure 1.1 shows a simplified version of the flow of funds for the 2018–2019 budget. A more up-to-date version will be issued for the more recent years which could show slight changes in the provision pathway.

The planned expenditure for NHS England by the Department of Health and Social Care has been set to increase by 3.4% annually to reflect the rise of healthcare costs and inflation in general.

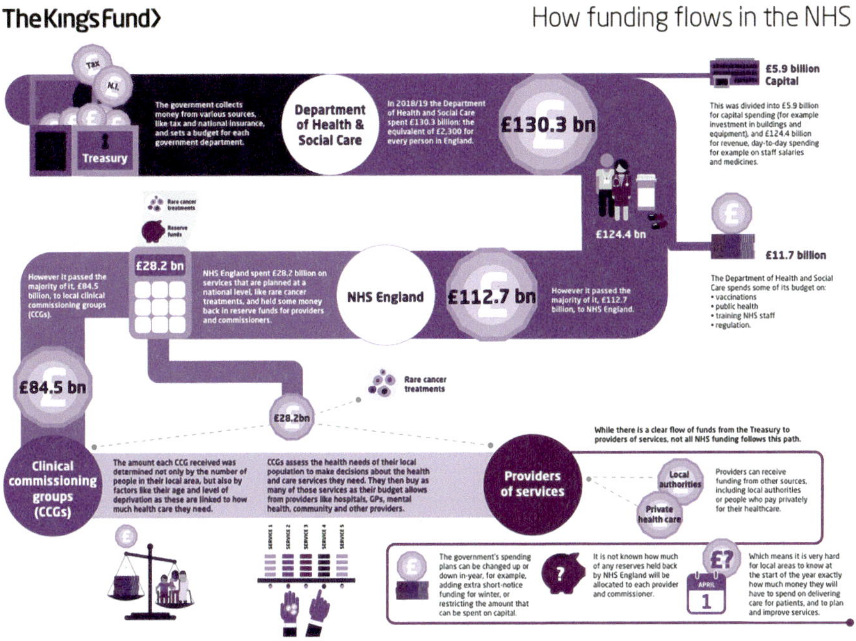


**Fig. 1.1** Flow diagram illustrating the flow of funds for 2018–2019 budget period. Reproduced with kind permission of The King's Fund (2020), UK. Available at: www.kingsfund.org.uk/audio-video/how-is-nhs-structured-funding-flow [accessed August 2022]

## 1.2 Organisational Structure of the Department of Health (DH)

The Secretary of State for Health and Social Care has the overarching responsibility for the DH. The DH is in turn made up of commissioning groups, healthcare services groups, monitoring and regulation groups, bodies that provide data and promote evidence-based medicine, and training and development bodies. The latest implementation, as mentioned above, starting from the first of July 2022 has been the introduction of ICSs which will act as the new commissioning groups at a local level (see Fig. 1.2).

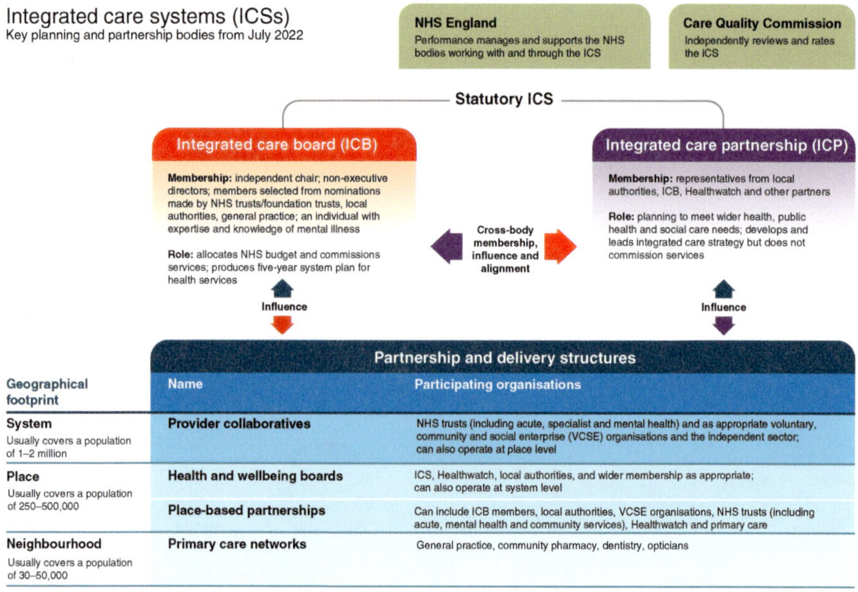


**Fig. 1.2** The introduction of ICSs to ensure optimal delivery of healthcare at a local level. Reproduced with kind permission of The King's Fund (2022), UK. Available at: https://www.kingsfund.org.uk/audio-video/integrated-care-systems-health-and-care-act [accessed September 2022]

### 1.2.1 Secretary of State for Health and Social Care

See: https://www.gov.uk/government/ministers/secretary-of-state-for-health-and-social-care

In addition to having overall responsibility for the work of the DH, the Secretary of State for Health and Social Care provides strategic leadership for public health, the NHS and social care in England, focusing on 5 key priorities:

- compassionate care,
- transparency,
- dementia,
- technology,
- better care.

### 1.2.2 Department of Health

See: www.gov.uk/government/organisations/department-of-health

The aim of the Department of Health (DH) is to improve the population's life expectancy and increase quality of life. The DH leads, shapes and funds health and social care in England. It ensures equal access to support, care and treatment. The DH outlines health policies and is accountable to Parliament with regard to the overall performance and public satisfaction with the health service.

### 1.2.3 NHS England

See: https://www.england.nhs.uk

Formerly known as the NHS Commissioning Group (before 2014), NHS England is responsible for:

- the majority of the healthcare budget,
- providing equal and fair access to healthcare,
- ensuring continuous improvement in treatment outcomes.
- preventing healthcare scandals such as that in mid-Staffordshire,
- placing patient interests first.

### 1.2.4 Clinical Commissioning Groups

See: www.nhscc.org/ccgs/

In April 2013, following the Health and Social Care Act (2012), NHS reorganisation led to the replacement of Primary Care Trusts (PCTs) with Clinical Commissioning Groups (CCGs).

The role of CCGs is to plan and commission healthcare services designed for a specific area or specialty to which they are assigned. There are currently 135 reduced from the original number 211. CCGs, with a catchment population of approximately 226,000 people per CCG. Members of CCG bodies include:

- hospital consultants,
- general practitioners,
- nurse practitioners,
- lay members.

CCGs hold approximately two-thirds of the total NHS England budget equivalent to £79.9 billion in 2019/2020.

The CCGs' responsibility lies beyond the primary care sector. They also commission secondary and tertiary care services such as:

- planned hospital care,
- rehabilitative care,
- urgent and emergency care (including out-of-hours),
- community health services,
- mental health and learning disability services.

On first of July 2022, CCGs have been superseded by ICSs or Integrated Care Systems. ICSs similarly to CCGs are responsible for providing healthcare in a specific geographic location. A total of 42 ICSs under the Health and Care Act 2022 have been statutorily tasked to deliver healthcare to clusters of population ranging in size from a minimum of 500,000 citizens to three million citizens.

Each ICS is governed by a board of executives and non-executives with 8 being the minimum; 5 executive and 3 non-executive directors.

The establishment of ICSs followed the launch of the document by NHS England entitled 'The NHS Long Term Plan' and consequently led to the closure of all CCGs.

### 1.2.5 National Institute for Health and Care Excellence (NICE)

See: www.nice.org.uk

NICE provides guidance on the best, most cost-effective and evidence-based treatment available. It was founded in 1999 and its role and responsibilities can be grouped into three main provision categories:

(a) provides guidance on:
  - therapeutical interventions by promoting evidence-based healthcare,
  - new technological advances in medicine by appraising them to ensure that only clinically effective procedures are introduced in the NHS,
  - existing technologies and diagnostics guidance,
  - interventional procedures,

(b) provides quality standards and performance benchmarks which are accomplished via:
  - Quality Standards.
  - Quality Outcomes Framework (QOF).
  - Clinical Commissioning Group Outcomes Indicator Set (CCGOIS).

(c) provides a wide range of supplementary information. This is disseminated via three platforms:
  - NICE Evidence (www.evidence.nhs.uk).
  - British National Formulary (BNF) and British National Formulary for Children (BNFC) (www.medicinescomplete.com/mc/bnf/current/ and. www.medicinescomplete.com/mc/bnfc/current/)
  - Medicines and Prescribing Support (www.nice.org.uk/about/nice-communities/medicines-and-prescribing).

### 1.2.6 NHS Improvement

See: https://improvement.nhs.uk

NHS Improvement is responsible for delivery of safe, high quality care within financially sustainable hospitals. NHS Improvement encompasses the following:

**Monitor**

See: www.monitor.gov.uk

Monitor, which used to be part of NHS Improvement since April 2016, is now no longer in existence. Monitor used to be an arm's-length body of the DH which regulated hospitals and foundation trusts. It monitored three key benchmarks of a trust:

- adherence to clinical governance principles and records serious breaches,
- clinical performance,
- financial performance.

Monitor used to be responsible for granting foundation status to trusts and for the overall quality of care provided and their financial performance. Monitor operated with an NHS provider licence. In 2015, Monitor merged with the NHS Trust Development Authority.

**NHS Trust Development Authority**

See: https://www.gov.uk/government/organisations/nhs-trust-development-authority

The NHSTDA aims to identify the specific needs of different trusts by providing support, restrain oversights and governance failures for all the NHS Trusts including small institutions in the community, primary care and secondary care to enable provision of high quality services.

NHSTDA is now part of NHS Improvement. See: https://improvement.nhs.uk. The main aim of NHS Improvement is to support NHS Foundation Trusts and ensure high quality healthcare provision.

**Patient Safety**

See: https://improvement.nhs.uk/improvement-hub/patient-safety/

Patient Safety encourages contact by patients to raise concerns or safety issues that they have experienced, or feel that they could prevent happening to themselves or to others. Patient Safety also manages incident reports filed through the National Reporting and Learning System (NRLS). Patient Safety encourages a safety culture within the NHS to eliminate the repetition of mistakes; this forms part of an improvement system that enables the delivery of high quality care.

**Advancing Change and Transformation Academy Team**

See: https://improvement.nhs.uk/resources/qsir-programme/

The Advancing Change and Transformation Academy Team [(ACTAT); previously Advancing Change Team) aims to deliver high quality programmes and masterclasses to healthcare clinicians and managers in institutions to help them redesign their services to improve them on a larger scale.

All ACTAT programmes are tailored to members at all levels within NHS institutions and are delivered by national and international experts. The programmes cover four key areas:

- leading transformational change,
- transformation essentials,
- quality, service improvement and redesign (QSIR),
- QSIR for the trainer.

**Intensive Support Teams**

See: https://www.nhsimas.nhs.uk/ist

Intensive Support Teams (ISTs) were incorporated in NHS Improvement on the first of April 2016; however, they are no longer in use.

They were historically composed of the following two groups:

- Elective Care—This team provides advice on how to manage demand, capacity and operational management in the elective care pathway. The aim is to reduce waiting times and improve access to community services.
- Emergency Care—This team's aim is to improve quality, safety and patient flow in A&E departments.

### 1.2.7 Health and Wellbeing Boards

See: https://www.local.gov.uk/our-support/our-improvement-offer/care-and-health-improvement/health-and-wellbeing-systems

Health and Wellbeing Boards (HWBs) act as a forum for local commissioners across the NHS, social care, public health and other services. The boards are intended to:

- increase democratic input into strategic decisions about health and wellbeing services,
- strengthen working relationships between health and social care,
- encourage integrated commissioning of health and social care services.

The ultimate aim of HWBs is to tailor the healthcare services to the local needs, thus targeting conditions more prevalent in specific geographic locations.

### 1.2.8 Care Quality Commission

See: www.cqc.org.uk

The Care Quality Commission (CQC) was founded in 2009 as an independent regulator of any health service provider in England. It was formed from three previous organisations: the Healthcare Commission, the Commission for Social Care Inspection and the Mental Health Act Commission. The CQC monitors, inspects and regulates services to make sure they meet fundamental standards of quality and safety; they publish what they find, including performance ratings, to help people choose care.

In the UK, the CQC:

- ensures that fundamental standards in daily practice in primary, secondary and tertiary care are met (see: www.cqc.org.uk/content/fundamental-standards).
- offers the public a register of listed practices that are CQC-approved.
- monitors, inspects and regulates care services.

- safeguards the wellbeing of vulnerable patients.
- listens and receives complaints from the public.
- involves the public on matters related to healthcare.
- pays attention to poorly performing practices to standardise services.
- carries out appropriate inspections and issues a licence to a healthcare provider after an on-site inspection. An inspection is usually carried out with 2 weeks of prior notice, although it can also be unannounced. The CQC has the authority to: issue a warning, restrict services, restrict admissions to the service, issue a penalty notice, suspend the provider's registration, cancel the registration and prosecute the provider in the case of illegal activity.

### 1.2.9 Public Health England

See: www.gov.uk/government/organisations/public-health-england

Public Health England (PHE) is an autonomous executive agency of the DH that advises and supports the government, local authorities and the NHS in a professionally independent manner. PHE provides national leadership and expert services to support public health, and also works with local government and the NHS to respond to emergencies. The main role of PHE is to protect and improve the nation's wellbeing, and reduce health inequalities.

PHE achieves its aims by:

- making the public healthier by encouraging discussions, raising awareness, advocating health campaigns, advising government and supporting action by local government, the NHS and other people and organisations.
- supporting the public so they can protect and improve their own health.
- protecting the nation's health.
- preparing for public health emergencies.
- sharing information and expertise with local authorities, industry and the NHS, to help them make improvements in the public's health.
- researching, collecting and analysing data to improve understanding of health and come up with answers to public health problems.
- reporting on improvements in the public's health so everyone can understand the challenge and the next steps.
- helping local authorities and the NHS to develop the public health system and its specialist workforce.

### 1.2.10 Other Important Organisations

**National Patient Safety Agency**

See: www.npsa.nhs.uk

The National Patient Safety Agency (NPSA) is an arm's-length body of the DH and its main role is to improve the safety and care of patients by informing, supporting and training healthcare workers, organisations and institutions. It does this by identifying and reducing risks to patients receiving NHS care at a national level.

The NRLS collects reports of patient safety incidents from all the trusts across England and Wales and identifies the risk of recurrence and consequences, thereby allowing the NPSA to help reduce the possibility of repeat incidences. In Northern Ireland, the HPSS, Health and Personal Social Services links to NRLS whilst in Scotland Health Improvement Scotland (HIS) through its improvement programmes ensures patient safety.

The Patient Safety division of NPSA works closely with the Royal Colleges, organisations, patient groups, strategic health authorities, NHS institutions, universities and research centres to promote patient safety.

**NHS Litigation Authority**

See: www.nhsla.com

The NHS Litigation Authority (NHSLA) provides funds for general and negligence claims against any NHS institution in England. It started operating in 1995 as a Special Health Authority. The NHSLA provides indemnity to NHS organisations and it shares lessons to be learnt at a national level to reduce future claims.

Legal and professional advice to the NHS and DH on equal pay and discrimination is also covered by NHSLA.

The Family Health Services Appeal Unit (FHSAU) is a branch of NHSLA which resolves contractual disputes between providers and their local commissioning bodies.

The National Clinical Assessment Service (NCAS) is an operating division and helps resolves concerns about healthcare professionals.

**Parliamentary Health Service Ombudsman**

See: www.ombudsman.org.uk

The Parliamentary Health Service Ombudsman (PHSO) is the organisation set up by, and responsible to, Parliament for processing complaints which were not managed at a local level. The legislation of the Parliamentary Ombudsman is drawn from the Parliamentary Commission Act (1967).

The PHSO's board has a maximum number of 13 members divided between executive and non-executive members.

The principles of the PHSO revolve around four main values: excellence, leadership, integrity and diversity.

The main role of the PHSO is to investigate complaints against trusts which might have been processed unfairly. It also helps patients who have received poor service from governmental departments and other public institutions. No investigations are undertaken by the PHSO unless the patient has processed the claim through the local (in the Trust) complaint system.

**Information Commissioner's Office**

See: https://ico.org.uk

The Information Commissioner's Office (ICO) regulates the adherence to the Freedom of Information Act, which gives any individual the right to access the personal information an organisation holds about them. The aim of the ICO is to ensure public openness of data belonging to patients or governmental bodies, including Trusts.

**The Royal Colleges**

See: the individual websites of each Royal College (Sect. 3.3).

The main aim of the Royal Colleges is to set standards for training of medical professionals and they undertake their role by setting national examinations (see Sect. 3.3 for more details).

## 1.3 Hospital Structures

Hospitals in the UK are responsible for providing secondary care medical services to a specified population within a geographical location.

They form part of a bigger group of providers totalling 217 known as NHS foundation trusts (FTs) and non-foundation trusts. Hospitals generally referred to as the Acute branch within this group offer services such as accident and emergency services (A&E), alongside acute medical and surgical services. The other groups include the following:

- Ambulance Trust which is responsible to stabilise patients and takes them to hospital.
- Community Trust which is responsible for covering a wide spectrum of care including home visits, treatment for minor injuries and outpatient services. They also offer outreach care to people enabling them to live independently.
- Mental Health Trust which is responsible for specialist psychological and psychiatric care, and work closely with primary and social care.

Hospitals are governed by a Board of directors whilst the day-to-day running of the clinical and non-clinical services is delegated to executive directors. A group of non-executive directors are also involved in managing the services and developing future plans and strategies.

Figure 1.3 shows a typical organisational arrangement in an NHS hospital in England.

NHS trusts are public sector bodies established by parliamentary order by the secretary of state for health to provide healthcare services to the NHS. They have a board of executive and non-executive directors, and are accountable to the secretary of state. There has been an expectation to regroup all NHS trusts as foundation trusts.

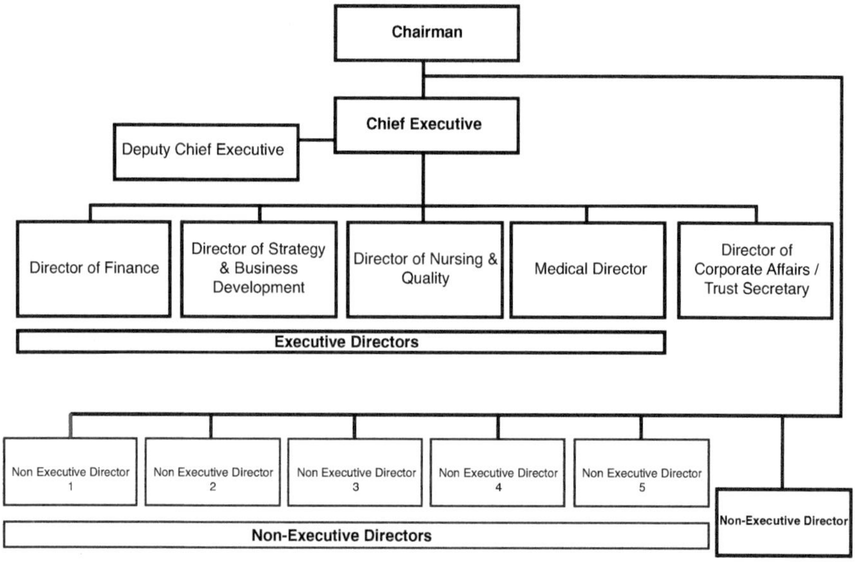


**Fig. 1.3** A simplified illustration of the management structure in a typical NHS hospital

NHS FTs represent trusts with a different legal status to NHS trusts with greater financial freedom, autonomy and local empowerment. They represent devolution of decision-making from central government to local communities. FTs are held accountable in a unique way. Local residents, staff, patients and service users can become members or governors, with the latter elected to closely follow the executive directors' performance. FTs in line with NHS trusts are also accountable to commissioners, the regulators and Parliament.

A differentiation between different type of hospitals within the secondary care sector lies in their affiliation with a local university. In such instances the hospitals forming part of an NHS trust or FT is referred to as a University Teaching Hospital (UTH). This demarcation allows a contrast between the latter and a District General Hospital (DGH) historically not affiliated to a university; however, this nowadays doesn't necessarily apply. The UTH designation in modern terms, refers to the shear size of the firms or departments with senior members of staff heaving a strong academic background. It also refers to a strong research background behind their overall activity. UTHs could be tertiary referral centres.

### 1.3.1 The Board of Directors

Made up of executive and non-executive members, the board of directors has collective responsibility for the performance of a Trust and exercises power on behalf of the Trust.

The board of directors is responsible for:

- setting the strategic direction of the Trust,
- monitoring performance against objectives,
- ensuring high standards of corporate governance,
- helping to promote links between the Trust and the local community.

***The Chief Executive and the Chairman*** The Chairman leads the Trust's board of directors and the Chief Executive leads all the executive directors. The non-executive directors are independent and do not take part in the day-to-day activities and decisions. They are mainly responsible for policy-making and planning exercises and although they are paid on a fee-basis, are not considered as employees. Non-Executive directors can also be appraised. They are also held to account by the Council of Governors.

**Executive Directors**
These are usually full-time members of staff and have responsibility for a specific area of the Trust's business. Typically, executive directors are appointed for the following directorates:

- Director of Nursing.
- Finance Director.
- Clinical Director.
- Director of Governance.
- Director of Workforce.
- Director of Operations and Strategy.

**Non-executive Directors**
The role of the non-executive directors is typically a supportive role to the executive directors and are not usually part of the Trust staff. Their role is not day-to-day management and is usually drawn from the local community following advertisement in the press. Their strategic role drives a trust's policy-making and planning exercises and are chosen based on their healthcare and management experience from previous employment. These board members utilise their external experience to offer an independent opinion to the board to assist with decision-making and overall management.

## Board Sub-Committees

Typically, a board of directors will also comprise various sub-committees, with each designed to take specific responsibility for a particular area and report back to the board to ensure that the highest standards of care are delivered. Typically sub-committees will be made up as follows:

- Audit committee: monitors aspects of financial reporting and risk management. It also collates internal and external audits, which are quality improvement exercises that seek to improve patient care and outcomes.
- Remuneration and appointments committee: monitors remuneration and terms of service of the executive directors. It also forms part of the panel to appoint executive directors.
- Quality and governance committee: monitors the quality of patient experience, safety and outcomes and ensures compliance with the standards set by external regulators.
- Finance and performance committee: monitors monthly reports on finance and operational performance to ensure targets are met.
- Equality and diversity committee: monitors equality and diversity issues relating to the services provided to patients, employment and procurement.
- Strategy committee: develops and sets plan for the Trust's future financial and healthcare plans.

## The Council of Governors

The main aim of the council of governors, who need to be elected individually, is to bring local accountability to the trust. They are not directors and occupy a non-paid position on a part-time basis. They do not usually form part of the trust's board committees although this could vary between trusts. The chair of the directors also chairs the council of governors.

The governors play important roles, such as appointing non-executive directors, and are an important part of the organisational structure of the Trust.

Governors are elected once a year for a minimum of 1 year and appointed in four areas:

1. Public governors: represent each of the local constituencies.
2. Patient governors: represent the Trust's patients.
3. Staff governors: represent a variety of staff roles across the Trust.
4. Nominated governors: appointed representatives of the Trust's stakeholder organisations, such as the local university.

If a governor moves from the geographical area he/she represents, his position would be presented for election.

The Council of Governors represent the views of the Foundation Trust and hold the Trust Board to account.

They also provide support and advice to the Trust to ensure:

- that the Trust delivers high quality care services.
- that the Trust provides high quality, effective and patient-focused services depending on the community needs.
- high standards of hospital governance and personal conduct.
- that there is public involvement in the trust.

The Council of Governors can also be encouraged to take a more executive role such as the appointment of external auditors. They also have a role regulating the Chairman and the non-executive directors of the Trust.

Governors are usually appointed for a three-year term but, subject to reappointment at the end of each term, can serve a maximum of nine years, although this can vary between different trusts.

The Council of Governors typically meets four or six times a year.

Typical Questions related to the structure of the NHS and different types of hospitals are found in boxes 1.1. and 1.2. below.

**Box 1.1 Differences between District General Hospitals (DGH) and University Teaching Hospitals (UTH)**

- A UTH is usually physically larger with a greater bed capacity and larger facilities.
- A UTH has a greater number of trainees, and a larger intake of junior doctors and doctors in specialty programmes.
- A UTH usually offers training programmes for allied health professionals.
- A UTH hosts a greater number of academic professionals.
- A UTH provides the majority of undergraduate training.
- A UTH can be part of an Academic Health Sciences Centre (AHSC).
- A UTH has a close link to a university.

**Box 1.2 The Essential Differences between an NHS Foundation Trust and an NHS Trust**

| | NHS Foundation Trust | NHS Trust |
|---|---|---|
| Government involvement | Board of Directors have autonomy on decisions affecting the trust | Central government is responsible for any decisions that impacts the trust |
| Financial regulation | Monitor | Trust development authority |
| Quality regulation | CQC | CQC |
| Financial independence | Board of directors make all the financial decisions | Trust board relays accountancy reports to central government |

## Further Readings

Department of Health (2015a) The government's mandate to NHS England for 2016–2017–mandate. www.england.nhs.uk/wp-content/uploads/2015/12/05.PB_.17.12.15-Annex-A-Mandate-to-NHS-England.pdf. Accessed December 2019

Department of Health (2015b) The NHS constitution for England–guidance. www.gov.uk/government/uploads/system/uploads/attachment_data/file/480482/NHS_Constitution_WEB.pdf. Accessed December 2019

Monitor (2012) NHS foundation trust governors and directors: working better together–documents and guidance. www.gov.uk/government/uploads/system/uploads/attachment_data/file/285965/Monitor_-_Director_govenor_interaction_report_June_2012_0.pdf. Accessed December 2019

Monitor (2014) Governance reviews for NHS foundation trusts–documents and guidance. www.gov.uk/government/uploads/system/uploads/attachment_data/file/294114/GovernanceReview14Jan13.pdf. Accessed December 2018

Monitor (2013) Your statutory duties–A reference guide for NHS foundation trust governors. https://assets.publishing.service.gov.uk/government/uploads/system/uploads/attachment_data/file/284473/Governors_guide_August_2013_UPDATED_NOV_13.pdf. Accessed January 2019

NHS England (2014) Understanding the new NHS–a guide for everyone working and training within the NHS–policy. https://www.nhs.uk/NHSEngland/thenhs/about/Documents/simple-nhs-guide.pdf. Accessed January 2019

# Quality, Efficiency and Value in the NHS

# 2

## 2.1 Introduction

Quality and efficiency are crucial for delivery of the best care possible through the continual striving to improve standards of care and reduce waste, of both manpower and financial resources.

In the NHS in England and Wales, this is obtained via QIPP: quality, innovation, productivity and prevention. In NHS Scotland, it is obtained via QIHUB: quality and innovation hub, and through quality and efficiency support team (QuEST); these support a number of programmes to improve the quality and efficiency of healthcare in Scotland.

QIPP sets an agenda rather than specific policies that need to be set in place and should be implemented in five target areas of medical care.

1. Commissioning and provision of healthcare—provision of NHS services involves:
   - primary care services,
   - NHS trusts and NHS foundation trusts, university teaching hospitals and specialised tertiary centres.
   - ambulance trusts,
   - mental health trusts,
   - community health trusts,
2. Health and wellbeing—the nation's overall health targets and wellbeing are addressed by Public Health England (PHE) and Health Well Being Boards (HWB). They implement policies, provide advice to the public and aim to decrease health inequalities. HWBs operate within local government authorities (LGA) and collaborate with local authorities to voice public concerns and aim to address local needs. HWBs promote partnership between NHS organisations, public health and government representatives at a local level and have no executive responsibilities. PHE is an executive agency of the Department of Health



S. Abela, *Leadership and Management in Healthcare*,
https://doi.org/10.1007/978-3-031-21025-9_2

and Social Care that works at a national level to improve the nation's heath and eliminate public health inequalities.

3. Regulation and monitoring—regulation is mainly conducted by:
   - NHS Improvement.
   - Trust Development Authority.
   - The National Quality Board.
   - The Care Quality Commission.
   - Healthwatch.
   - Professional monitoring by the councils, with the key ones being:
   - The General Medical Council (GMC).
   - The General Dental Council (GDC).
   - The Nursing and Midwifery Council (NMC).
   - The General Pharmaceutical Council (GPhC).
   - The General Optical Council (GOC).
   - The Health and Care Professionals Council (HCPC).
4. Education and training—Health Education England (HEE), an independent arm's-length body of DH with a budget of £4.07 billion for 2019/2020, is responsible for education and training. HEE provides:
   - planning and succession planning for the healthcare workforce,
   - the structures for medical training,
   - funding for NHS education and training,
   - and promotes innovation in healthcare delivery,
   - appoints and collaborates with Local Education and Training Boards (LETBs).

     There are 13 LETBs and their main aim is to provide training for both clinical and non-clinical staff. LETBs are sub-committees of HEE and they structure training based on needs locally.
5. Leadership and management—all health professionals should participate in leadership and management to continuously drive an improvement in the quality of care provided. Leadership and management is delivered through:
   - the NHS Leadership Academy which is part of the NHS with the principal aim of providing excellent leadership throughout the whole NHS organisation by delivering leadership programmes, tools and models.
   - The Faculty of Medical Leadership and Management which supports medics and dentists by providing schemes and networks to guide them in obtaining leadership skills and delivering efficient policies.

## 2.2 Quality in the NHS

Quality in the NHS is centered around clinical effectiveness, patient safety and patient experience. This focus ensures that the NHS delivers the highest level of care possible. These areas of focus have been outlined in the NHS Outcomes Framework which comprises five domains:

Domain 1: preventing people from dying prematurely.
Domain 2: enhancing quality of life for people with long-term conditions.
Domain 3: helping people to recover from episodes of ill health or following injury.
Domain 4: ensuring people have a positive experience and can recommend the service to family and friends (the 'family and friends' test).
Domain 5: providing a safe environment out of harm's way.

Domains 1 to 3 provide clinical effectiveness whilst domains 4 and 5 provide a good experience and safety for the patient.

### 2.2.1 NHS Improvement Quality

See: https://webarchive.nationalarchives.gov.uk/20160805121830/http://www.nhsiq.nhs.uk/

NHS Improvement Quality (NHSIQ) was established in April 2013 and was the driving force in improving the quality of care provided by the NHS. The latest objectives of NHSIQ for 2014/2015, before being superseded by the NHS Sustainable Improvement Team (NHS SIT) in 2016 (see Sect. 2.2.2) included the following:

- providing new ideas and innovations in healthcare,
- developing the professionals' skills, knowledge and infrastructure,
- reducing mortality from chronic disease,
- improving the quality of life for people with long-term conditions,
- adopting 7-day services,
- supporting the delivery of recommendations from the Urgent and Emergency Care (UEC) Review,
- improving the patient experience,
- improving patient safety,
- providing strategies that allow the NHS to cope with unexpected and urgent matters.

### 2.2.2 NHS Improvement (NHSI)

See: https://improvement.nhs.uk

NHSI is a non-departmental public body formed on the first of April 2016 and since the same date in 2019, NHS England and NHS improvement have been combined as a single organisation. NHSI's constituents include seven regional teams representing different geographical regions within England principally: East of England, London, Midlands, North East and Yorkshire, North West, South East and South West.

Their main driving force to deliver the NHS Long Term Plan. Seven integrated teams each catering for a specific geographical area play a leadership role in ensuring the best support systems in place via sustainability and transformation partnerships (STPs) and integrated care systems (ICS).

Sustainability and Transformation Partnerships (STPs): Formed In 2016, this partnership is a joint effort between NHS organisations and local councils. Their aim is to coordinate, collaborate and plan the improvement of the residents' day-to-day health.

Integrated Care systems (ICS): ICS is an even closer collaboration between the NHS and local councils with the aim of streamlining and ensuring lean management of the resources available at a local level to improve the delivery of NHS care.

**The Five Year Forward View**

See: www.england.nhs.uk/futurenhs/

The Five Year Forward View, a document outlining the NHS strategic planning was first published in October 2014. It outlined the new models of care on which the NHS is based. The original document was developed by partner organisations and recommended changes to the future of NHS delivery to reduce health inequalities and improve overall longevity. It set out a vision based on seven new models of care:

Multi-speciality community providers.
Primary and acute care systems.
Urgent and emergency care networks.
Acute care collaborators.
Specialised care.
Modern maternity services.
Enhanced health in care homes.

The measures have been reviewed in the 'Next steps on the NHS Five Year Forward View' publication, first published on the 31st of March 2017 and later updated on the eighth of March 2019.

This updated plan aimed at recognising realistic challenges that faces the NHS and ways to overcome them and prioritise the aspects of care which needed improvement the most.

### 2.2.3 Commissioning for Quality and Innovation

See: https://www.england.nhs.uk/nhs-standard-contract/cquin/

CQUIN is a framework within the NHS that aims to improve the efficiency of healthcare delivery by rewarding the achievement of improvement targets in healthcare. Its intention is to drive a positive transformation of the NHS in its entirety including the patients, the providers, and the staff.

NHS England usually publishes an annual CQUIN guidance document, with the latest publication being 2020/21 CQUIN.

The most recent CQUIN document outlines four key areas listed below that will support the fulfilment of the Long Term Plan:

- Prevention of ill health.
- Mental Health.
- Best practice pathways.
- Patient safety.

### 2.2.4 Quality Premium

See: www.england.nhs.uk/resources/resources-for-ccgs/ccg-out-tool/ccg-ois/qual-prem/

QP is a scheme that rewards CCGs for any improvements they accomplish in the delivery of their services. The QP guidance document is published annually, but for the first time the latest document extends the scheme for 2 years and so covers 2017–2019.

The maximum QP payment is £5 per head of population and 85% of QP is based on five national targets, each with a 17% weighting:

- Early cancer diagnosis.
- GP access and experience.
- continuing healthcare,
- mental health,
- bloodstream infections.

The rest of the 15% is left to the discretion of the local CCG and is based on the local needs and health inequalities.

The QP can be reduced if CCGs fail to meet four waiting time standards that form part of the NHS Constitution requirements:

1. Maximum 18 weeks from referral to treatment.
2. Maximum 4 hour waits in A&E departments.
3. Maximum 2 month (62 day) wait from urgent GP referral to first definitive treatment for cancer.
4. Maximum 8 minute response for Category A ambulance calls.

### 2.2.5 Healthcare Quality Improvement Partnership

See: www.hqip.org.uk/about-us/

HQIP is an independent organisation led by the Academy of Medical Royal Colleges, the Royal College of Nursing, and National Voices. It also welcomes feedback from other stakeholders to reflect the current state of healthcare provision. The aim of HQIP is to promote quality in healthcare and share results from clinical audits for the benefit of the healthcare providers.

### 2.2.6 National Voices

See: www.nationalvoices.org.uk

National Voices is a coalition of healthcare charity organisations that represent public opinion and raise concerns about any deficiencies in a particular geographical area. National Voices also represent the voluntary organisations that provide an essential service in health and social care.

### 2.2.7 National Confidential Enquiry into Patient Outcome and Death

See: www.ncepod.org.uk/ncepod.html

The work undertaken by NCEPOD is commissioned by HQIP on behalf of NHS England. The main aim of NCEPOD is to improve the quality of care provided by assessing the overall management of patients. They obtain data by undertaking confidential surveys and rendering their results accessible for common use.

### 2.2.8 Quality and Outcomes Framework

See: www.nhsemployers.org/your-workforce/primary-care-contacts/general-medical-services/quality-and-outcomes-framework

QOF is a scheme available to GPs which rewards them for achieving clinical targets which promote high quality care. All QOFs are available in the guidance paper '2019/2020 General Medical Services contract Quality and Outcomes Framework'.

Payments are made at the end of the financial year, with all monetary awards being based on a formula. The ratio of the actual achievement to the potential achievement is multiplied by the number of points available for the indicator and the monetary value for each QOF point.

### 2.2.9 National Quality Board

See: www.england.nhs.uk/ourwork/part-rel/nqb/

The aim of the NQB is to raise the standard of healthcare provision and increase the quality of service provision at a national level. It provides coordinated leadership for quality on behalf of the following national bodies: Department of Health, Public Health England, NHS England, CQC, NHS Improvement and NICE.

### 2.2.10 Patient Reported Outcome Measures

See: www.england.nhs.uk/statistics/statistical-work-areas/proms/

PROMs is another quality-centred initiative that focuses on measuring the improvement in a patient's quality of life, for four surgical procedures:

- hip replacements,
- knee replacements,
- groin hernia,
- varicose veins.

The PROMs scheme started in 2009 and is reported by NHS providers through self-completed questionnaires.

## 2.3 Efficiency Models in Healthcare

The NHS has continuously invested a sizeable portion of its budget on efficiency models, including the current Conservative government. These models and their implementation is complex and provides a challenge to all the personnel involved.

To date, several models have been designed in an attempt to render healthcare providers more efficient and so reduce waste. One of the ways of ensuring efficiency is to promote organisational development. Qualitative and quantitative studies have been performed to identify the most beneficial model to adopt. The following models provide NHS organisations with methods to embrace change and develop to ensure improved efficiency in their operations.

This section examines the commonly applied models in healthcare and describes their application in the NHS; some of these models have been adopted from other industries, but healthcare staff should, nevertheless, be familiar with them.

### 2.3.1 The Lean Model

The lean model originated in the car industry and has also been used successfully in other industries, but its basic principles can equally be applied in healthcare delivery. Successful outcomes entail the utilisation of the lean model throughout the whole organisation. The aims of this model are to improve efficiency and eliminate unnecessary procedures. The model is based on the following five principles.

1. Specify value—in healthcare, value to the patient would be translated as minimal time in the waiting room, perfect outcomes and no adverse effects.
2. Identify and visualise the value stream (patient journey)—in healthcare, a patient's procedure has to be streamlined and efficient. In ideal circumstances, at the time of diagnosis the patient has the necessary investigations carried out, followed shortly thereafter by the procedure.
3. Make the process and value flow—in healthcare, this implies a smooth process between the referral centres and the different institutions needed to treat the problem. If the diagnosis has been completed by the GP, one referral to the trust should initiate the process for completion of the procedure.
4. Letting the customers "pull"—in healthcare, this would imply that the patients are the main driving force. For example, if a hospital department is aware of a

referral being sent, the department should be ready to contact the patient and book him/her for treatment.

5. Pursue perfection—in healthcare this would equate to patients receiving the best possible care with the best possible outcomes and no adverse effects.

### 2.3.2 McKinsey 7S Framework

The McKinsey 7S Framework (see Fig. 2.1) is an organisational development model developed to increase a system's efficiency. It is based on the need to align seven internal elements of an organisation, which are often be grouped as follows:

1. Hard factors consisting of strategy, structure and systems.
2. Soft factors consisting of shared values, skills, staff and style.

For an organisation to perform well, the model requires that all seven elements are aligned and mutually reinforcing. The model can therefore be used to help identify what needs to be realigned to improve performance, or to maintain performance during change.

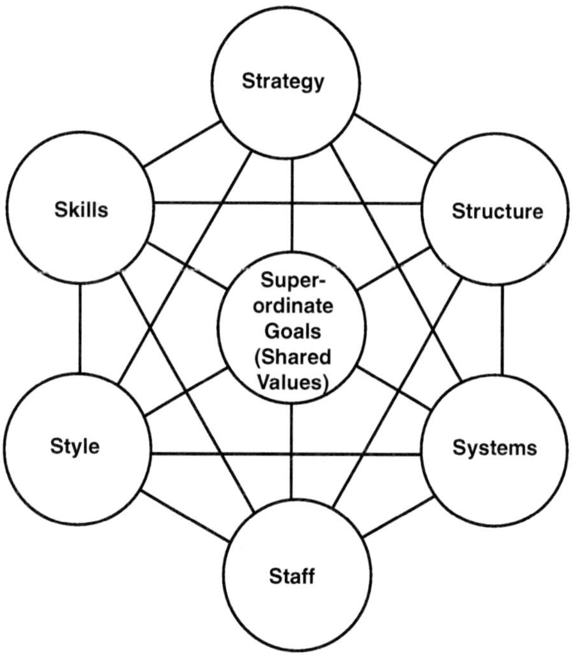


**Fig. 2.1** The McKinsey 7S Framework showing the interrelationship between the seven internal elements of an organisation. Figure reproduced from http://en.wikipedia.org/wiki/McKinsey_7S_Framework and is reproduced here under a CC 2.5 licence. The model originally appeared in: Waterman, Peters and Phillips (1980) Structure is not organisation. McKinsey Quarterly, in-house journal. McKinsey & Co., New York

### 2.3.3 Kotter's 8-Step Change Model

Managing changes to keep an organisation thriving involves planning, designing and implementing strategies; however, almost everything revolves around managing staff. Kotter created the 8-Step Change Model (see Fig. 2.2) to lead change in an organisation. This model's 8 steps are listed below:

1. Establish urgency—in healthcare, leaders should inspire all NHS staff and motivate them to undertake the actions necessary for change.
2. Build a coalition—this involves selecting the right professionals that match the job specification with the right emotional commitment, and the right professional skills mix.

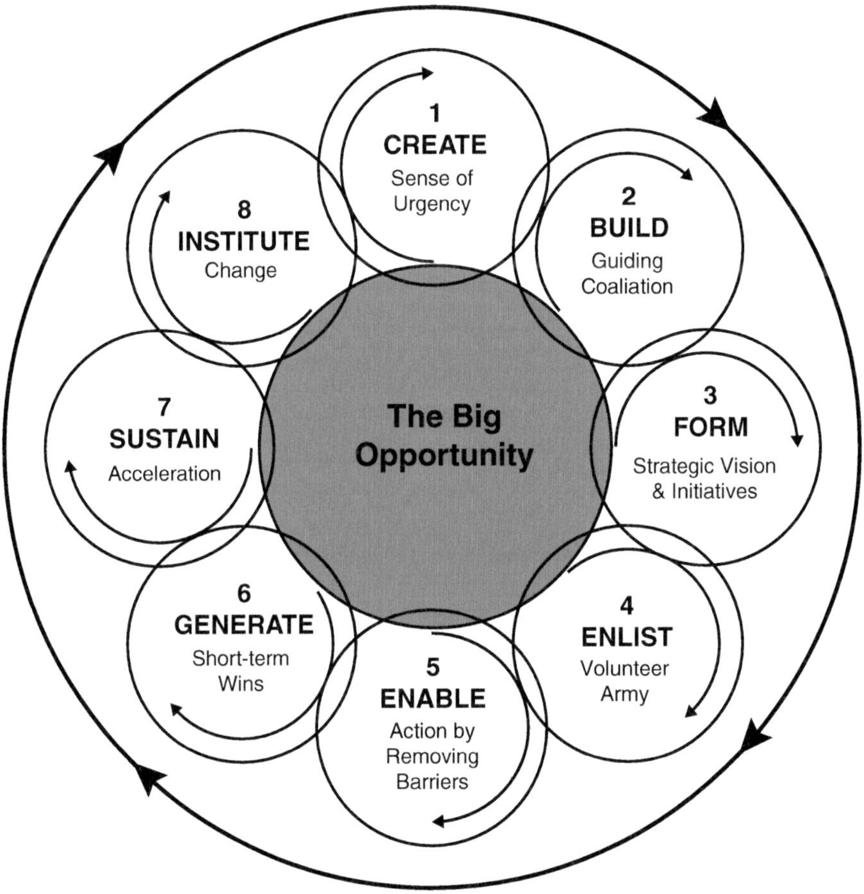


**Fig. 2.2** Kotter's 8-Step Change Model showing the cyclical process of managing change. Figure reproduced with permission from Kotter International, Cambridge, Massachusetts, USA and attribution by Pkor43 at English Wikipedia, CC BY-SA 3.0 http://creativecommons.org/licenses/by-sa/3.0/, via Wikimedia Commons

3. Form strategic vision and initiatives—leaders should specify the Trust's targets (CQUIN and QP targets) and make the mission statement common knowledge.
4. Enlist a volunteer army—the whole team should comprise individuals who are willing to improve the organisation. Regular meetings and staff participation exercises help create a sense of team-belonging.
5. Enable action by removing barriers—eliminate any obstacles that could be detrimental to bringing about change. Ensure that all team members are aware of the NHS's aims and objectives.
6. Generate short-term wins—the NHS should consistently monitor and track all the SMART aims set, i.e. those aims which are: specific, measurable, achievable, reasonable and time-specific.
7. Sustain acceleration—the management teams should change or eliminate any old policies that could slow down the process of change. Staff that are fundamental to the organisation should be promoted and new staff identified to continuously strengthen a successful network.
8. Institutional change—the NHS should ensure the identification of successful behaviours in staff and put in place strategies to ensure staff with similar attributes are selected in future.

### 2.3.4 Lewin's Change Management Model

One key aspect which makes organisations successful is the ability to adapt to the demands of the sector and/or clients. A successful organisation meets such demands by adapting and introducing change rapidly and effectively.

The model introduced by Lewin is based on three phases, as shown in Fig. 2.3.

The first phase, the unfreeze phase, refers to the phase in which the staff in an organisation are readied to accept the change, understand the reason for the changes recommended, and are willing to overcome the inbuilt inertia associated with an organisation's traditional mindset.

The second phase, the change phase, is where the staff are implementing the new systems and the organisation is adapting (often a period of transition and confusion), before staff embrace the benefits of the new systems and help to motivate colleagues.

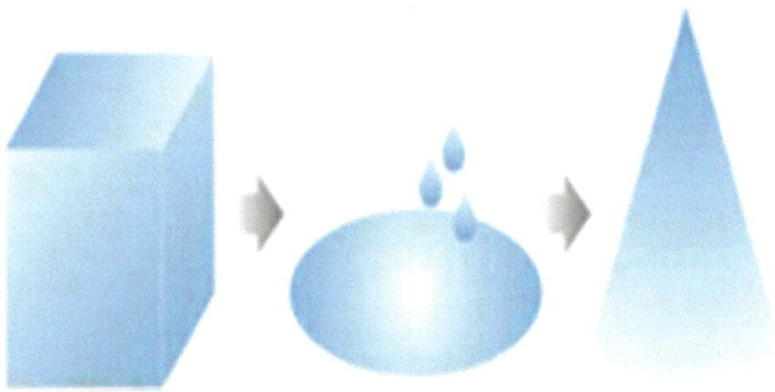

**Fig. 2.3** The three phases of Lewin's Change Management Model. This was reproduced by kind permission of Mind Tools

The third phase, the freeze phase, is when the employees, staff and the whole organisation have fully embraced the changes and its effects are seen throughout the whole hierarchy of staff who are all now comfortable with the changes implemented.

### 2.3.5 The Congruence Model

This change management model, first described by Nadler and Tushman in 1989, identifies weak areas within the organisation by focusing on its performance which is believed to be dependent on four elements:

1. Tasks.
2. People.
3. Structure.
4. Culture.

Higher compatibility between these four elements results in a more efficient and productive organisation, hence the name Congruence Model.

Applying the Congruence Model involves three fundamental steps or stages:

The first stage: Analysis of each of the above-mentioned elements; the task or work, the members of staff, the organisational structure and finally the culture.

The second stage: Analysis of the relationship between the elements; work and staff, work and structure, structure and staff, staff and culture, culture and work and structure and culture.

The third stage: Identify the incompatibilities identified by the stages 1 and 2, identify solutions to overcome them, sustain and build congruence.

### 2.3.6 The Burke–Litwin Model

This model was described by Litwin and Burke in 1992 and is based on 12 key drivers of change:

1. External environment.
2. Mission and strategy.
3. Leadership.
4. Organisational culture.
5. Structure.
6. Management practices.
7. Systems.
8. Work unit climate.
9. Task and individual skills.
10. Individual needs and values.
11. Motivation.
12. Individual and organisational performance.

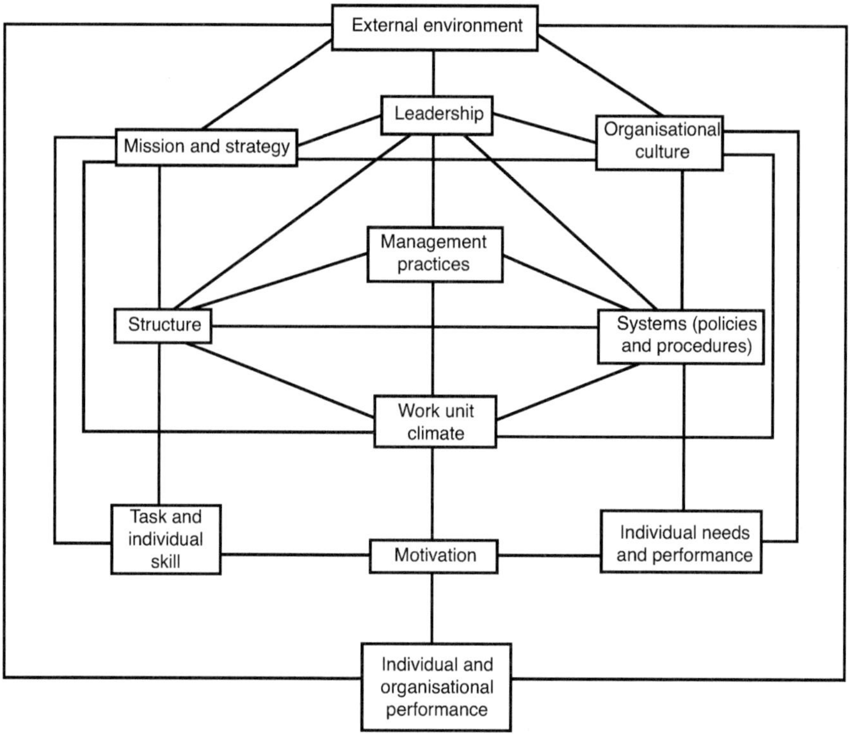


**Fig. 2.4** The Burke–Litwin Model for change management. Figure reproduced with permission of SAGE Publications from Burke and Litwin (1992) 'Causal Model of Organisational Performance and Change', Journal of Management. © 1992

The Burke–Litwin model (Fig. 2.4) shows these various drivers of change and ranks them in terms of importance, with the most important factors featuring at the top of the diagram. The lower layers become gradually less important. The model argues that all of the factors are integrated (to greater or lesser degrees) and so a change in one will eventually affect all other factors.

The model suggests that most change can be traced back to external drivers for change. In a wider scope, external environmental factors can entail market, legislative or economical changes within an organisation. Specifically in healthcare, examples of such external environment can include a change in the legislative manner of how a hospital is managed such as a change in its status from a trust to a foundation trust. This would affect the daily management and accounting of the organisation. Another example that could be representative of an external environmental change is a change in the monetary revenue scheme. Such a change could involve a switch from block contracting where a hospital get its activity paid in bulk at the start of a financial year to payment by results (PbR), where the hospital would be paid based on the activity carried out throughout the year.

### 2.3.7 Weisbord's Six-Box Model

This model, developed by Weisbord in 1976, aims to assess the functionality of an organisation. In contrast to the Burke–Litwin model, Weisbord's model looks at the internal issues and his six-box model comprises the following components:

## 2.4 Purpose

1. Structure.
2. Relationships.
3. Rewards.
4. Leadership.
5. Helpful mechanisms.

Weisbord's model provides a diagnostic framework, analysing not only the individual elements highlighted above but also the interrelationship between them. Weisbord's model divides the analytical approach into:

- Formal—the official stance taken by the organisation in the form of official documentation and policies.
- Informal—looks into the 'on-ground' or actual events employed by staff members.

The purpose component allows clarification of the organisation's goals, aims and objectives whilst the structure component looks into the appropriateness of the organisation's structure to deliver its scope of practice.

The relationship component examines the interrelationship between different individuals within a department and between departments. An existential mechanism improves any disputes and facilitates quick resolution of matters leading to increased efficiency.

Reaping rewards, honours and benefits whilst simultaneously outlining potential repercussions for inappropriate action places an organisation at a productive advantage.

Leadership is key in this model and is placed in a central position in Fig. 2.5 below, highlighting its importance. An organisation's leader/leaders should be able to merge the individual efforts and promote the organisation's purpose, values, integrity and principles.

Finally, the helpful mechanisms component refers to the systems in place to improve the implementation and facilitate delivery of the organisation's goals.

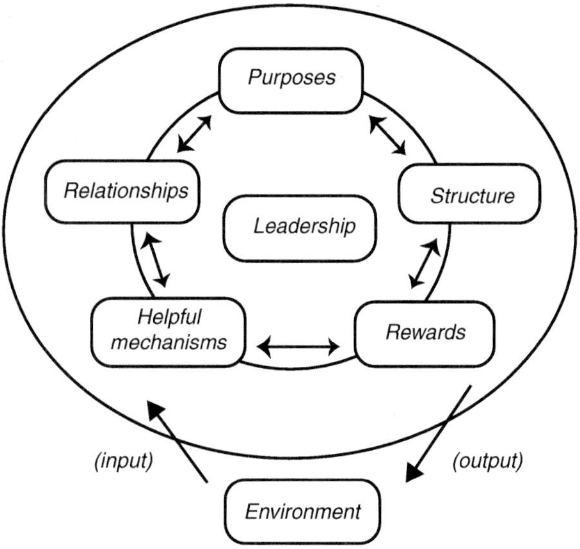


**Fig. 2.5** Weisbord's Six-Box Model. Reproduced with permission of SAGE Publications from Weisbord (1976). 'Group and Organisation Management, Organisational Diagnosis: Six Places to Look for Trouble with or without a Theory' 1976. Group and Organisation Management. © 1976

## Further Readings

Burke W, Litwin GH (1992) A causal model of organisational performance and change. J Manag 18:523

Department of Health (2016) Operational productivity and performance in English NHS acute hospitals: unwarranted variations–an independent report. www.gov.uk/government/uploads/system/uploads/attachment_data/file/499229/Operational_productivity_A.pdf. Accessed December 2018

Institute for Healthcare Improvement (2005) Going lean in health care. IHI Innovation Series white paper, Cambridge, MA

Nadler DA, Tushman ML (1983) A congruence model for organisational assessment. In: Lawler EE, Nadler DA, Cammann C (eds) Organizational assessment: perspectives on the measurement of organizational behavior on the quality of work life. Wiley, Chichester

National Quality Board (2016) Shared commitment to quality–guidance. www.england.nhs.uk/wp-content/uploads/2016/12/nqb-shared-commitment-frmwrk.pdf. Accessed December 2018

NHS Employers (2019/20) General medical services (GMS) Contract: quality and outcomes framework (QOF)–Guidance for GMS contract 2019/20 in England https://www.england.nhs.uk/wp-content/uploads/2019/05/gms-contract-qof-guidance-april-2019.pdf. Accessed December 2019

NHS England (2014) Understanding the new NHS www.nhs.uk/NHSEngland/thenhs/about/Documents/simple-nhs-guide.pdf. Accessed December 2018

NHS England (2016) Commissioning for quality and innovation–guidance for 2017–2019. https://www.england.nhs.uk/wp-content/uploads/2018/04/cquin-guidance-2018-19.pdf. Accessed January 2019

NHS England (2020) Commissioning for quality and innovation–guidance for 2020–2021. https://www.england.nhs.uk/wp-content/uploads/2020/01/FINAL-CQUIN-20-21-Core-Guidance-190220.pdf. Accessed January 2021

NHS England (2019) The NHS long term plan. https://www.longtermplan.nhs.uk/wp-content/uploads/2019/08/nhs-long-term-plan-version-1.2.pdf. Accessed January 2021

NHS England (2017) Next steps on the NHS five year forward view. https://www.england.nhs.uk/wp-content/uploads/2017/03/NEXT-STEPS-ON-THE-NHS-FIVE-YEAR-FORWARD-VIEW.pdf. Accessed January 2021

NHS Institute for Innovation and Improvement (2010). The handbook of quality and service improvement tools. http://www.miltonkeynesccg.nhs.uk/resources/uploads/files/NHS%20III%20Handbook%20serviceimprove.pdf. Accessed December 2018

Weisbord MR (1976) Organisational diagnosis: six places to look for trouble with or without a theory. Group & Organisation Studies 1:430

# 3 Evidence-Based Practice in the NHS

## 3.1 Introduction

There has been a huge drive for clinicians to adopt an evidence-based approach in their everyday practice. Evidence-based practice (EBP) sometimes referred to as evidence-based medicine (EBM) is an approach to practice which allows clinicians to optimise their decisions using evidence from high quality research, ideally from systematic reviews, randomised controlled trials and meta-analyses. Using this evidence will provide the patient with the best possible, and previously proven, treatments.

High quality evidence provides a clinician with increased knowledge and the evidence should be acquired through continuous education and obtaining guidance at three different levels.

- Local level—guidelines for practice are readily available from a trusts' intranet, as are clinical and managerial policies. Wherever you work in the NHS, you should make sure you are familiar with the local guidelines.
- National level—guidelines are produced and updated regularly by NICE (National Institute for Health and Care Excellence) and also many of the Royal Colleges. Other sources include SIGN (Scottish Intercollegiate Guidelines Network) and the Centre for Reviews and Dissemination.
- International level—a source of high quality evidence for medicine is available through Cochrane (previously The Cochrane Collaboration), a global independent network of scientists, healthcare professionals, medics and other health stakeholders that collates the most recent evidence, all free from commercial bias. Other international databases including collections of meta-analyses, systematic reviews, randomised controlled trials and internationally peer-reviewed journals: MEDLINE, Embase, CINAHL, PsycINFO and PubMed.



S. Abela, *Leadership and Management in Healthcare*,
https://doi.org/10.1007/978-3-031-21025-9_3

## 3.2 NICE

NICE was established in 1999 and was originally known as the National Institute of Clinical Excellence, before joining with the Health Development Agency in 2005 and, in 2013, changing its name to the National Institute for Health and Care Excellence when it became a non-departmental public body. The Department of Health (DH) sponsors all NICE activities; however, it remains an independent entity.

The main role of NICE is to issue guidelines in four areas:

- Clinical practice guidelines.
- Social care services and procedures.
- Health technology appraisals within the NHS.
- Public health promotion and ill-health avoidance.

The NICE Board, which sets the strategic priorities and policies, comprises executive and non-executive directors. All appointments to the NICE Board must be made in accordance with the Code of Practice for Ministerial Appointments to Public Bodies. The executive directors are responsible for day-to-day decision-making and issuing of the body's policies and strategies, whilst the non-executive directors have an advisory role.

NICE is structured into 7 main subdivisions.

1. Centre for Guidelines (CfG).
   The CfG arm of NICE issues clinical guidelines, public health guidelines and social care guidelines. It is responsible for the promotion of good health, prevention of disease and providing the most appropriate type of treatment for specific disease and delivery of social care.
2. Centre for Health and Social Care Directorate.
   This directorate is responsible for:
   - quality standards,
   - medicines and prescribing programme,
   - the British National Formulary (BNF),
   - the accreditation advisory committee,
   - the Fellows and Scholars Programme,
   - the Public Involvement Programme,
   - the NICE field team,
   - the NICE Pathways,
   - the implementation of guidance,
   - the Health Technologies Adoption Programme (HTAP),
   - the student champion scheme,
   - shared learning,

3. Centre for Health Technology Evaluation (CHTE).
   The CHTE develops guidance on the use of new medicinal products, innovations, techniques and interventional procedures. It is also responsible for The Patient Access Scheme Liaison Unit (PASLU), a platform bridging pharmaceutical companies and patients, which assesses the feasibility of new drugs being made available to NHS patients.
4. Centre for Communications Directorate.
   This communicates NICE guidance and disseminates new publications. It also manages press and public enquiries and hosts the NICE website.
5. Science, Evidence and Analytics Directorate.
   This directorate is responsible for updating the science and evidence available to update its policies and recommendations. It is also responsible for:
   - Science policy and research.
   - EUnetHTA and international collaboration.
   - Special scientific projects.
   - Research recommendations.
   - Information services.
   - Evidence services.
   - UK PharmaScan.
   - Healthcare Database Advanced Search (HDAS).
   - Evidence Search.
   - Intellectual property and reuse of NICE content.
   - Data and analytics.
6. Finance, Strategy and Transformation Directorate.
   This directorate manages all NICE services such as financial, business planning, human resources, corporate governance and its estates and facilities.
7. Digital, Information and Technology Directorate.
   This directorate is responsible for the design, the development and maintenance of NICE digital operations. It is also responsible for the upkeep of the internal guidance production systems and the IT operations and infrastructure.

## 3.3 NICE Decision Making

Given the wider scope of public healthcare provision, NICE cannot simply qualify all type of newly launched medicines. Its aim is to review the clinical and economic evidence, and make recommendations and issue guidance on the most appropriate use of both new and existing medicines and/or devices.

Occasionally, exceptions can be made, and a single treatment can be reviewed in isolation however most often than not, NICE evaluates all the current treatments for a particular condition, including more contemporary ones against gold standard practices which have a strong evidence-based background and issues recommendations on the most-cost-effective approach.

NICE as a decision-making entity is required to account for both the scientific evidence and thus clinical effectiveness together with the cost-effective thus justifying the implementation or purchase of a new medicine or technology. The first step in considering new medicines by NICE is to consider the health benefits.

### 3.3.1 Clinical Effectiveness

The first stage of any consideration process of a new intervention is the evaluation of the scientific evidence available. An independent academic group is commissioned to review this together with a public consultation. An appraisal committee is also formed to consider all the issues related to this new intervention. The data appraised can be in the form of experimental or observational studies; however, systematic reviews and meta-analyses are the preferred sources of data.

During the consideration process, NICE considers above all the robustness of data available, the direct comparisons to current methods of treatment, the reported improvement in quality of life, the validity and real-world efficacy of the proposed treatment.

### 3.3.2 Cost-Effectiveness

NICE's preferred measure of cost-effectiveness is the incremental cost-effectiveness ratio (ICER). This compares the increased health gain measured as quality-adjusted life year (QALY) to the increased costs. It also considers the savings attributable to the introduction of the new medicine or technology. In essence, NICE equates the increase in perceived QALY and the increased costs. In case of a positive finding, NICE needs to justify the introduction to the existing practices.

### 3.3.3 Social Value Judgements

NICE's final decision is always made official and published justifying the introduction of a new medical product or technique to society at large. This is referred to as distributive justice. This exercise ensures optimal use of public funds to the benefit of the society in its entirety.

In case of justification at an individual level, NICE considers a case-by-case approach.

NICE's advisory bodies make a judgement based on an ICER of between £20,000 to £30,000 per QALY. Consequently, NICE's advisory bodies would be unlikely to reject, an intervention that costs less than £20,000 per QALY as it is considered as cost-effective. On the other hand, an intervention which costs more than £20,000 to £30,000 per QALY is likely to be rejected.

NICE additionally can also make special allowances and considerations to individual situations that could benefit from an intervention that could exceed £20,000 to £30,000 per QALY threshold.

### 3.3.4 Implementing a New Practice

As mentioned earlier in this chapter, NICE's advisory bodies reach conclusions after very thorough considerations and the robustness of the procedures involved, allows its advisory bodies to encourage medical professionals to follow the guidelines issued.

Ultimately, at a clinical level, the decisions and clinical judgements remain within the clinicians' remit. The local commissioners and healthcare providers tasked with economic modelling and increasing cost-effectiveness across the healthcare platform will invariably be guided by the recommendations made available by NICE and make adherence to them a priority.

**Example 1**

For contextual purposes, a specific healthcare commissioner in a specific geographical area is considering the introduction of planned caesarean section (CS) deliveries to increase cost-effectiveness and safety.

NICE's role in this case is to issue a guidance that will be available for:

- Healthcare professionals outlining the basis for their decisions.
- Commissioners and providers to outline the most-cost-effective method of delivery in this case.
- Public health and trust managers to enable evidence-based knowledge backing the procedure that they offer.
- Public at large, in this case, pregnant women and their families.

For approval purposes, the findings reported by NICE have to show that the benefits of CS in comparison to normal delivery are consistently greater and the outcomes are excellent with less frequent morbidities and/or complications. This will allow NICE to justify the widespread introduction of this intervention and encourage medical professionals to recommend this procedure.

In this instance, NICE did produce a guidance and also provided a summary with regard to the benefits of CS over normal delivery which is kept updated to reflect the latest scientific evidence. The clinical guideline, CG132, published on the 23rd of November 2011 and updated on the fourth of September 2019 provided the conclusions listed in box 3.1 below.

**Box 3.1. Summary of Clinical Guideline CG132**

*Planned caesarean section may reduce the risk of the following in women:*

- *pain in the area between the vagina and anus (perineum) and in the abdomen (tummy) during birth and 3 days afterwards,*
- *injury to the vagina,*
- *heavy bleeding soon after birth,*
- *shock caused by loss of blood.*

*Planned caesarean section may increase the risk of the following in babies:*

- *intensive care unit admission.*

*Planned caesarean section may increase the risk of the following in women:*

- *longer hospital stay,*
- *bleeding after the birth that needs a hysterectomy (removal of the womb),*
- *heart attack.*

The above information will allow all the medical professionals and providers alike with the necessary information on which to base their decisions.

More detailed information together with a summary and a patients' version of these effects is always made available for professional and public use alike. In this case, this information can be found in appendix C of the NICE guideline, available from:

*www.nice.org.uk/CG132*

All the NICE published guidelines can be readily accessible online via the NICE website: www.nice.org.uk/guidance

**Example 2**

A novel drug is available for the prevention of chronic migraine called Erenumab, produced by Novartis which has been accepted by the U.S. Food and Drug Administration. This drug, a new class that works by blocking a molecule involved in migraine attacks has to be evaluated by NICE with regard to its cost-effectiveness and the economical feasibility of prescribing it to chronic migraine patients.

In this example, NICE first establishes the indications for the use of the new drug Erenumab, which is prevention of chronic and recurrent migraine in adults totalling a minimum of four times a month with the use of three failed attempts with existing medication. NICE then examines the cost per patient which in this case is £5000 per patient per year and also compares its efficacy to existing medication and the current evidence behind the use of the new drug.

NICE review showed that there was no evidence in the reported trials of preventative measures undertaken and could not prove superiority to the already NICE-approved botulinum toxin type A. Because of these reasons NICE could not approve the widespread use of Erenumab as acceptable nor cost-effective.

The final draft of this guidance has been published on the 26th of September 2019 and the final appraisal document is available online: https://www.nice.org.uk/guidance/gid-ta10302/documents/appraisal-consultation-document

Continuous updates will ensure that new scientific evidence can be factored in and the guidance modified or altered as needed.

## Further Readings

NICE (2011) Caesarean section: clinical guideline https://www.nice.org.uk/guidance/cg132/resources/caesarean-section-pdf-35109507009733. Accessed January 2021

NICE (2014) Developing NICE guidelines: the manual–process and methods www.nice.org.uk/process/pmg20/resources/developing-nice-guidelines-the-manual-pdf-72286708700869. Accessed December 2019

NICE (2018) Erenumab for preventing migraine; appraisal consultation document https://www.nice.org.uk/guidance/gid-ta10302/documents/appraisal-consultation-document. Accessed January 2021

# Healthcare Regulation in the UK

# 4

## 4.1 Introduction

All healthcare professionals aspiring to practice in the UK have to join the General Medical Council (GMC) in the case of doctors. Other types of healthcare professionals have to register with their respective regulatory body depending on the nature of their profession.

There are ten health and social care regulatory bodies overseeing the adequacy of the 'register' by ensuring that the professionals listed are all adhering to the required standards.

The main responsibilities of a regulator include:

- Setting standards of competence, conduct and ethical behaviour
- Setting a uniform expected level of knowledge and skills
- Maintain and update a register for professionals and public use
- Investigate any malpractice or incidents that could lead to a compromise to public safety

All the regulators in the UK are regulated by the Professional Standard Authority for Health and Social Care whose activity is in turn regulated by Parliament. The Privy Council consults the authority on the annual budget needed and this sets the fees that the regulators must pay. The Health Committee can be made accountable for their work.

## 4.2 The Royal Colleges

The Royal Colleges are professional membership organisations responsible for setting standards within their specialty and for supervising the training of doctors in the UK and abroad. They relay information of a doctor's progress to the General Medical

 
S. Abela, *Leadership and Management in Healthcare*,
https://doi.org/10.1007/978-3-031-21025-9_4

Council (GMC) or General Dental Council (GDC); see section 4.3.2 and 4.3.3 below for more details on these two organisations. It is the GMC and the GDC who two ultimately authorise registration and eligibility to practise as a doctor or a dental surgeon. Other commonwealth countries have adopted Royal Colleges with a similar role.

There are 17 medical and surgical Royal Colleges in the UK, listed alphabetically below:

- The Royal College of Anaesthetists
- The Royal College of Emergency Medicine
- The Royal College of General Practitioners
- The Royal College of Nursing
- The Royal College of Obstetricians and Gynaecologists
- The Royal College of Ophthalmologists
- The Royal College of Paediatrics and Child Health
- The Royal College of Pathologists
- The Royal College of Physicians
- The Royal College of Physicians and Surgeons of Glasgow
- The Royal College of Physicians of Edinburgh
- The Royal College of Psychiatrists
- The Royal College of Radiologists
- The Royal College of Speech and Language Therapists
- The Royal College of Surgeons of Edinburgh
- The Royal College of Surgeons of England
- The Royal College of Veterinary Surgeons

The Royal Colleges are registered charities that rely financially on membership fees. Members are principally clinicians, physicians or surgeons. The principal role of the Royal Colleges is the advancement of medical and surgical standards and improved care for patients.

Other roles of The Royal Colleges include the following:

- Supervision of trainee doctors including helping with the provision of the necessary evidence of training.
- Providing courses and training for medical professionals.
- Providing examinations to maintain the highest standards in medicine and surgery.
- Promoting research and disseminating findings, including of audit projects.
- Providing advice to trusts by nominating a regional college advisor.
- Acting as an advisory body for other governmental and non-governmental institutions.
- Preserving historical and contemporary medical and surgical knowledge.
- Forming international collaborations.
- Facilitating dialogue between members of the public and the medical profession.

## 4.3 Health and Social Care Regulators

There are 10 health and social care regulators in the UK (in alphabetic order):

- General Chiropractic Council (GCC)
- General Dental Council (GDC)
- General Medical Council (GMC)
- General Optical Council (GOC)
- General Osteopathic Council (GOsC)
- General Pharmaceutical Council (GPhC)
- Health and Care Professions Council (HCPC)
- Nursing and Midwifery Council (NMC)
- Pharmaceutical Society of Northern Ireland (PSNI)
- Social Work England (SWE)

These regulators are responsible for protecting the public and ensuring adherence to the relevant standards they set. All professionals involved in national or private health and social care should be registered with a regulator and failure to adhere to the registration is illegal and the individual can be prosecuted. All of the regulators are in turn regulated by the Professional Standards Authority for Health and Social Care, previously known as CHRE (Council for Healthcare Regulatory Excellence).

### 4.3.1 The General Chiropractic Council

See: www.gcc-uk.org

The GCC is an independent statutory body accountable to the Parliament with the sole aim of regulating chiropractors, registering the practising chiropractors and ensuring the highest standards within the profession.

The jurisdiction of GCC spans the whole of the UK and currently registers three thousand five hundred professionals.

In line with other regulators the GCC:

- Promotes standards
- Develops the profession
- Investigates and acts
- Delivers value

The values and access of the body are valid for patients and public, the registered professionals and stakeholders equally.

### 4.3.2 The General Dental Council

See: www.gdc-uk.org

The GDC is a fee-based charitable organisation that registers all dental surgeons in the UK. It maintains standards for dental professionals through nine core principles:

- Places patients first.
- Communicates effectively.
- Provides valid consent to patients.
- Maintains and protects patients' information.
- Has a clear and effective complaints procedure.
- Works well with colleagues.
- Maintains, develops and works within your professional knowledge and skills.
- Raises concerns if patients are at risk.
- Does not put the profession's reputation at risk.

The GDC now comprises 12 council members and the Chief Executive team; the structure was changed in October 2013 when it previously consisted of 24 council members.

The Chief Executive team comprises the following directors:

- human resources
- finance and corporate services
- policy and communications
- regulation
- governance

### 4.3.3 The General Medical Council

See: www.gmc-uk.org

The GMC is a fee-based charity which is responsible for registering all practicing medical professionals in the UK. Its legal basis is covered by the Medical Act 1958 and it has a statutory obligation to the Privy Council which in turn is answerable to the House of Commons.

The GMC has four core principles:

- Excellence
- Fairness
- Transparency
- Collaboration

The role of the GMC in the UK is as follows:

- Assessing overseas doctors' undergraduate and postgraduate training equivalence to the training programmes in the UK.
- Managing the medical register.
- Investigating poorly performing doctors (see also Box 3.1).
- Revalidation.

The GMC comprises 12 members (6 lay and 6 medical), all appointed following an independent appointment process.

### 4.3.4 The General Optical Council

See: www.optical.org

The GOC regulates the optical professionals in the UK. This encompasses the following:

- Optometrists
- Dispensing opticians
- Student opticians
- Optical businesses

The GOC's board has 12 members and eight committees, three of which are non-statutory. They include the following:

- Audit and Risk Committee
- Remuneration Committee
- Nominations Committee

The other five committees are statutory and have been defined under the Opticians Act and related Rules:

- Companies Committee
- Education Committee
- Investigation Committee
- Registration Committee
- Standards Committee

The Council's Fitness to Practise and Registration Appeals Committee are populated by independent hearings panel members.

### 4.3.5 The General Osteopathic Council

See: www.osteopathy.org.uk

The GOsC's main responsibility is to regulate the osteopathic profession and its activity. It protects above all and promotes public safety. It also maintains and ensures adherence to the profession's standards.

The GOsC consists of six committees and a small team of staff members. The committees include the following:

- The investigating committee
- The policy and education committee
- The professional conduct committee
- The health committee
- The audit committee
- The remuneration and appointments committee

The staff members, part of the senior management team are accountable to the chief executive and are as follows:

- The registrar
- The Director of education, standards and development
- The Director of fitness to practise
- The Registration and resources team
- The Communications and engagement team
- The Secretariat

### 4.3.6 The General Pharmaceutical Council

See: www.pharmacyregulation.org

The GPhC is the statutory regulator for pharmacists, pharmacy technicians and pharmacies in the UK. The role and functions of the GPhC are set out in Pharmacy Order, a legislative framework.

The GPhC council consists of fourteen members: seven pharmaceutical professionals and seven members of the public. It is constituted of seven committees; three are non-statutory and four are statutory.

Non-statutory committees:

- Audit and risk committee
- Remuneration committee
- Appointments committee
- Finance and planning committee

Statutory committees:

- Investigating committee
- Fitness to practice committee
- Appeals committee

### 4.3.7 The Health and Care Professions Council

See: www.hcpc-uk.org

The HCPC's main aim is to set standards and keep an up-to-date register of fifteen health and care professionals. The council also takes actions if public safety is a concern.

The inclusion of the health and care professionals includes the following in alphabetical order:

| | |
|---|---|
| • Arts therapists | • Orthoptists |
| • Biomedical scientists | • Paramedics |
| • Chiropodists/podiatrists | • Physiotherapists |
| • Clinical scientists | • Practitioner psychologists |
| • Dietitians | • Prosthetists/Orthotists |
| • Hearing aid dispensers | • Radiographers |
| • Occupational therapists | • Speech and language therapists |
| Operating department practitioners | |

The council consists of twelve members: six registrants and six members of the public. The appointments to the Council are all made via the Privy Council.

HCPC is constituted of seven committees that advise and assist the council:

- The audit and risk assurance committee
- The education and training committee
- The people and resources committee
- The education and training panels
- The remuneration committee
- The former committees
- The professional liaison groups

### 4.3.8 The Nursing and Midwifery Council

See: www.nmc.org.uk

The NMC is the professional regulator for nurses and midwifes in the UK and nursing associates in England.

The NMC Council is made up of twelve members: six members of the public and six professionals. All members are appointed by the Privy Council.

The council has three committees which assists the council:

- the audit committee
- the remuneration committee
- the investment committee

### 4.3.9 The Pharmaceutical Society of Northern Ireland

See: www.psni.org.uk

The PSNI is an elected and representative body, made up of pharmacists representing all aspects of the pharmacy profession in Northern Ireland. The PSNI seeks to develop the pharmacy profession in Northern Ireland, by representation and leadership, with the public interest as its main priority.

The Council consists of up to fourteen members: seven registrants and seven members of the public. Council members are appointed on a competency basis by the Department of Health, Social Services and Public Safety, DHSSPS for periods of between 2 and 4 years.

The council is assisted by the following committees:

- The Resources committee
- The Audit and Risk committee
- The Corporate Communications committee
- The Education, Standards & Registration committee
- The Fitness to Practise Committee

### 4.3.10 The Social Work England

See: www.socialworkengland.org.uk

Social Work England is the regulator for social care workers in England. Established by the Social Workers Regulation 2018, is a non-departmental, arm's-length body from the government.

Social work England is constituted by eight board members appointed through the public appointments process and two committees:

- the Audit and Risk Committee and,
- the Remuneration Committee

## 4.4 Requirements for Practising Medicine in the UK

Application for a medical position requires the possession of a licence to practice. The latter is issued by the GMC and automatically enlists a doctor for the revalidation process every 5 years. Licencing was introduced in 2009 whilst revalidation was introduced in 2012. A list of medical practitioners with a valid licence can be found online: www.gmc-uk.org/doctors/register/LRMP.asp (accessed December 2018). Doctors can be found on two possible registration lists: the GP Register or the Specialist Register (for doctors who have undergone further training in one specialism).

A doctor can be registered with the GMC but not possess a valid licence. Registration will entitle a doctor to practise with restrictions such as providing emergency care, provide 'good samaritan' acts. Registration is also needed if a doctor wants to pay a reduced annual GMC retention fee, works abroad and is unsure if he/she will return to practice in the UK, or want to prove current or past good standing with other regulators.

The fees to cover an application for full registration and annual retention are both £425.

New and overseas applicants and doctors restoring the registration after a period of absence can benefit from the Approved Practice Settings (APS) scheme. This scheme provides guidance and supervision, where appropriate, supplemented with regular appraisals to provide doctors with the appropriate training for optimal care delivery. The APS scheme provides the clinician with a designated body to ensure progress and effective delivery of care but it does not limit the doctor to practise within the designated body only.

### 4.4.1 Provisional Registration

Purpose: provide registrant enough time (12 months) to obtain recognised training in a formal programme to allow progress to full registration. The maximum length of provisional registration is 3 years and 30 days. If application to full registration is not approved, a registrant can't reapply for a provisional registration. Further support can be obtained from the LETB.

Recognised programmes: year 1 of the Foundation programme (FY1). Following completion of FY1, a Certificate of Experience is issued which complements the authorisation by the LETB, providing the necessary evidence to obtain full registration.

### 4.4.2 Registration for Doctors with European Qualifications

Medical graduates from the EU or the EEA member states are governed by EC rights which allows citizens to move freely within the same zone. This EC right does not automatically authenticate registrants and they still need to undergo the application procedure.

All applicants need to demonstrate English language capability and this is done through the International English Language Test System test which must be passed in the 2 years prior to registration.

### 4.4.3 Registration for Doctors with International Qualifications

Internationally qualified doctors applying for registration require the following:

- An acceptable medical degree—the primary medical degree has to originate from an institution recognised by the GMC; these are listed on the World Directory of Medical Schools or on the International Medical Education Directory. The GMC specifically lists the qualifications that are not accepted by country of origin (see www.gmc-uk.org/doctors/registration_applications/14390.asp—accessed December 2018).
- English language capability—a valid IELTS certificate which is less than 2 years old and has an overall score of at least 7.5 (with a score of 7.0 in the speaking, listening, reading and writing tests). A registrant is exempt from sitting the IELTS if he/she has a valid medical degree less than 2 years old that was taught in English. IELTS is not needed for prospective registrants where English is the first and native language, or they have already been accepted for employment by a UK organisation.
- Previous registration and licencing history—the applicant should give details of previous registrations and licences held in other countries, detailing the start and end dates for verification.
- Certificates of good standing—these should be from medical authorities or institutions to which the applicant has been affiliated.
- Knowledge and skills—the applicant should show the following:
  - a pass score in PLAB—note that since September 2017 this is only valid for 2 years.
  - certificates of acceptable postgraduate qualifications.
  - certificates of approval for sponsorship by an approved sponsor.
  - certificate of completion of specialist training or general practitioner training.
- Work experience and previously held posts—a minimum of 12 months of continuous medical training in both medicine and surgery have to be undertaken to allow eligibility for full registration. This is also known as internship.

## Further Readings

Department of Health (2015) Pharmaceutical price regulation scheme 2014 – guidance. www.gov.uk/government/publications/pharmaceutical-price-regulation-scheme-2014. Accessed Dec 2019

GMC (2013) The good medical practice framework for appraisal and revalidation. www.gmc-uk.org/static/documents/content/The_Good_medical_practice_framework_for_appraisal_and_revalidation_-_DC5707.pdf. Accessed Dec 2019

Health Care and Associated Professions (2010) The pharmacy order 2020. https://www.legislation.gov.uk/uksi/2010/231/pdfs/uksi_20100231_en.pdf. Accessed Jan 2021

# Staffing in the NHS 5

## 5.1 Introduction

Staffing and the workforce is one of the most important elements of the NHS. Hiring the appropriate number of employees with the correct skill mix is key to improving the quality of care provided by the NHS and increasing the efficiency of delivery of that care.

Safe care is a core principle of the NHS. NHS England is continuously working on safe staffing to reduce harm at the point of delivery by partnering with other stakeholders such as NICE, Monitor, Health Education England and CQC amongst others. NICE have also issued separate guidance recommending the ideal ratios of nurses and midwives to inpatients.

## 5.2 Recruitment

The NHS remains one of the largest employers in the world and currently employs over one million and three hundred thousand staff. With these figures, it is important that not only robust recruitment systems are in place but they are also tailored to the unique needs of a department or fulfil the needs of a specific sector.

Nevertheless, the increase in awareness, longer life expectancies and better medical technology demands an ever increasing demand on staff numbers and it is estimated that the NHS requires approximately eighty to eighty-five thousand members of staff of which fifty thousand should be registered nurses.

With regard to general medical practitioners the current estimated shortfall is of two thousand five hundred; however, this could increase to seven thousand in approximately five years time.

A publication by NHS England entitled "We are the NHS: People Plan 2020/21 - action for us all" highlights the strategies laid out to manage this human resources shortfall.



S. Abela, *Leadership and Management in Healthcare*,
https://doi.org/10.1007/978-3-031-21025-9_5

The plan together with a complimentary policy, "Our NHS People Promise" set out a fully detailed strategy on how this implementation will take place.

Below is a detailed account of the enrolment of Consultants within the NHS, as together with the other members of the team they form an important part of a department's fabric.

## 5.3 Role of Consultants in the NHS

Hospital consultants provide an invaluable service across the NHS and are responsible for the daily running of departments. Employment of a consultant is a very carefully planned procedure due to both the financial implications and also the additional resources needed, such as auxiliary staff and equipment to complement and support the newly appointed consultant. The application process is initiated via an official submission of a business plan and acceptance by the hospital's management. Consultants develop systems of care and provide the managerial expertise by combining the right skill mix for excellent clinical care.

### 5.3.1 Summary of the Key Roles of an NHS Consultant

NHS consultants' roles and clinical responsibilities are overseen by the Medical services head at the employing hospital.

1. Clinical
   - Provides complex clinical care and manages the most difficult clinical scenarios autonomously and with competence.
   - Provides and runs multidisciplinary teams for those patients who need clinical input from more than one specialty.
   - Has ultimate responsibility for patients admitted to his or her firm/team.
2. Managerial
   - Quality assures the team's performance and puts measures in place to continuously improve outcomes.
   - Promotes and introduces innovative techniques in the department.
   - Implements guidelines produced by a trust, the relevant Royal Colleges and NICE.
   - May assess and appraise junior doctors, trainees and consultant colleagues.
3. Research
   - Shares new knowledge at a local, national and international level.
   - Conducts primary and secondary research to boost medical knowledge.
4. Teaching
   - Provides clinical supervision, and didactic teaching to undergraduate and postgraduate medical students, junior doctors and less experienced colleagues.
   - Holds continuous professional development sessions for the whole team.

5. National Health Service
   - NHS consultants are usually involved at a local level and form part of the local area's framework and local NHS organisations, such as managed clinical networks, to improve healthcare provision and meet local demands.
6. Public health
   - Engages in public health meetings to discuss future provision of treatment to meet the demands of the population.

## 5.4 Job Planning

Job planning is the process by which an employer sets out for the employee (doctor in this case), their individual duties and responsibilities. Job plans are prospective and are essentially an agreement between employee and employer.

The aim of the job planning process is to ascertain that workloads are appropriately balanced and suited to the needs of the department.

A job plan is usually presented in weekly terms. The consultant contract was reviewed in 2003 and the new contract states that the ideal ratio is 7.5 direct clinical care (DCC) sessions to 2.5 sessions supporting professional activity (SPA). However, acute trusts are moving towards a ratio of 8 DCC to 2 SPA sessions. Electronic logging of doctors' hours, using software such as Zircadian, formerly known as HealthMedics, allows trusts to job plan sessions more precisely.

### 5.4.1 Direct Clinical Care and Supporting Professional Activities

DCC sessions can involve any of the following activities:

- Administration, such as booking appointments
- Consultation or new patient clinics
- Day surgery
- GP/GDP communication
- Histopathology/radiological reporting
- Inpatient operating
- Inpatient ward round
- Interventional radiology
- Own patient treatment session
- Patient administration
- Patient referral writing
- Patient/relative communication
- Direct undergraduate or postgraduate clinical supervision

SPA sessions can involve any of the following:

- undergraduate or postgraduate-related activities such as preparation for assessments, vivas or clinically related examinations
- audit projects
- research
- job planning/appraisals
- departmental meetings
- clinical management team meetings
- journal club/educational meetings
- CPD-related activities
- mandatory and statutory training
- local clinical governance meetings
- local/national committee meetings

Activities in general can be categorised as follows:

- Direct Clinical Care (DCC)
- Supporting Professional Activity (SPA)

Other duties such as the duties listed below are categorised separately; however, they are allocated to the job plan to allow the necessary time and resources to implement them:

- Additional NHS
- Responsibilities External Duties
- Fee paying services
- Private Professional Services
- Medical School Services

What comes first: revalidation or job planning?

Job planning should always come first. This is carried out by the clinical lead within the same department. The job planning has to be revised annually and is a separate entity from the appraisal and revalidation. The appraisal, discussed in the next section, in case of a trainee is carried out by the trainee's educational supervisor who might not necessarily be the line manager or clinical lead.

## 5.5 Appraisals

**What Is an Appraisal?**

An appraisal is a process essential for revalidation and should provide documentary evidence of the clinical, educational, managerial and research skills acquired over the previous year by the doctor. The appraisal should ascertain that a doctor is progressing in line with the GMC's 'Good medical practice' principles (see: www.gmc-uk.org/guidance/good_medical_practice.asp).

**Who Carries Out the Appraisal?**

An appraiser, usually the clinical lead of a department or a senior colleague within the same specialty. It should be a two-way process between the appraiser and the clinician being appraised.

In the case of GPs, appraisers are trained individuals with suitable experience; they are not employed within the same practice. The appraisers do not need to be involved in practice or in full employment. NHS England lays out core training criteria and follow-up obligations to maintain registration as an appraiser. Appraisers are monitored and supported by an administrative team and an appraisal lead. The appraisal process is dynamic and establishes continuous improvement and evidence of dedication to medicine and its advances. A GP who is uncomfortable with their allocated appraiser has the right to demand a change of their appraisal.

**The Responsible Officer (RO)**

The RO, responsible officer is an individual within an organisation that is responsible at renewing the medic's validation. The employing institution would in turn support the appraisal and validation.

The RO is usually the Deputy Medical Director and acts as a mediator for approving the doctor's revalidation between NHS bodies and the GMC, excluding any limiting factors which might mean that the appraisal process should be investigated further or postponed.

The RO can issue three types of recommendations:

1. Positive recommendation
2. Deferral
3. Non-engagement

In case of a deferral, further information might be needed for the RO to upgrade his recommendation. In case of a non-engagement outcome, the medic would have failed to show an active role and participation in the revalidation process.

ROs for GPs are usually within the NHS England Local Area Teams (LATs); however, the same process is applied.

An updated list of designated bodies, ROs with the relevant contact information can be found online on the GMC's website or by following this link: https://www.gmc-uk.org/-/media/documents/DB_list_with_RO_details___DC3503.pdf_52637845.pdf—accessed January 2019.

The website is updated every 3 weeks and when accessed the last update is found on the top of the list.

The annual appraisal process is used to check for satisfactory evidence of up-to-date knowledge and fitness to practice, and to establish that there are no outstanding investigations or concerns.

How often is the appraisal process carried out?

Each doctor should have an appraisal every 12 months.

Why is the appraisal process important?

Information collated by the clinician being appraised

↓

Appraiser uses 5 scoring system;
unacceptable, below average, good, outstanding and unable to comment

↓

Medical Responsible Officer (from the same trust) evaluates and shares information with Medical Director
(assuming the Responsible Officer and Medical Director are not the same person)

↓

Medical Director evaluates information obtained

↓

Recommendation to the clinician being appraised

**Fig. 5.1** The appraisal process

Appraisal is a professional developmental process that allows doctors to identify learning needs and to ensure they are working productively and in line with the priorities and requirements of the organisation in which they practise.

It also allows doctors to formulate a personal development plan (PDP) which in turn allows completion of the appraisal and directs the practitioner to undertake the necessary courses to adhere to the appraisal guidelines.

What constitutes an appraisal process?

The appraisal process is illustrated in Fig. 5.1. Each trust provides its own version of the appraisal form; however, it always contains four main sections:

1. Background details—confirmation of personal details such as current residential address, marital status, etc.
2. Details of medical activities—review of the job plan and details of daily and weekly commitments in relation to DCC and SPA sessions.
3. Supporting documentation and the previous year's report—detailed account of progress achieved in four key areas:
   - Knowledge, skills and performance—each clinician should be continuously monitoring his/her personal performance, demonstrating improvement in overall performance, and applying knowledge to daily practice.
   - Safety and quality—each clinician should demonstrate awareness of safety principles and policies set to minimise risk.
   - Communication, partnership and teamwork—each clinician should demonstrate effective communication with colleagues, senior members of staff and patients, in addition to showing commitment to teaching and supporting more junior members of staff.

- Maintaining trust—demonstrate respect to patients, putting their dignity first, and applying the Equality and Discrimination Act rules to avoid discrimination.

  The supporting documentation should include multi-source feedback (MSF) from 10–15 colleagues reviewing the doctor's performance and interaction with the whole team. This should be structured by obtaining feedback from a range of colleagues, including clinicians from other departments, nursing officers, complementary staff such as radiographers, secretarial personnel, and other members of staff not necessarily involved directly in patient care. This makes the MSF reflect as many qualities of the doctor being appraised as possible.

4. Summary of appraisal—this should include a revised PDP and agreed action for the forthcoming year.

## 5.6 Revalidation

Revalidation, which was introduced in 2012, is the process (see Fig. 5.2) through which the GMC confirms that a doctor is eligible to continue to practise and so renews their licence. The revalidation process takes place every 5 years and the process is in addition to annual appraisal. Every doctor has an organisation which delivers both the appraisal and revalidation.

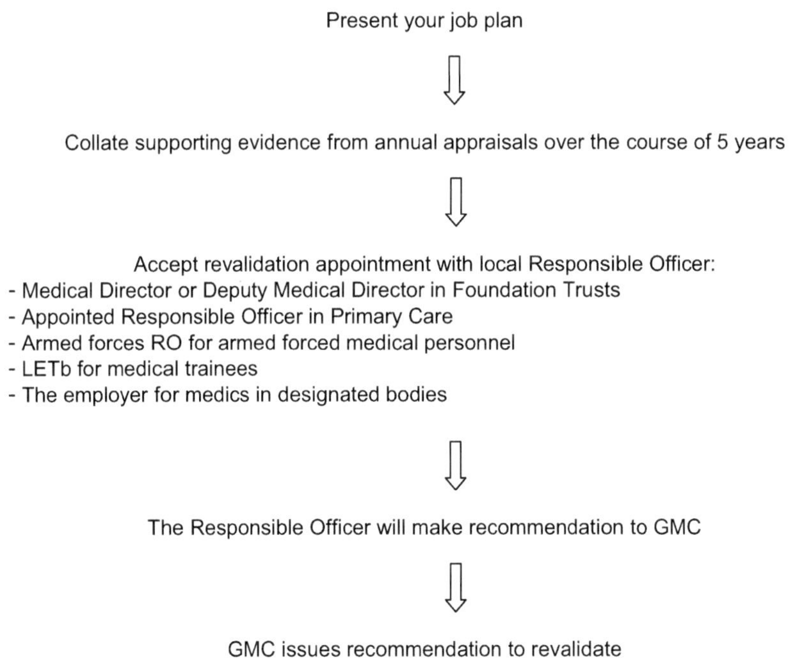


**Fig. 5.2** The revalidation process

What is the process of revalidation?

The revalidation process has four main elements:

- Reflection by the doctor being appraised on current practice.
- Identification of improvements that could be undertaken.
- Reflection on continuing professional education the doctor has undertaken.
- Demonstration of fitness to practice.

Who is the appraiser and the responsible officer?

The appraiser, chosen by the organisation providing the employment, is invariably a senior member of staff within or outside the department, whilst the responsible officer is usually the Medical Director of the organisation (or another director delegated by the medical director, usually the deputy medical director).

What documents should you prepare prior to revalidation?

There are six types of supporting information required:

1. Continuing professional development (CPD)—CPD comprises formal and informal learning activities. This provides evidence that the doctor has undergone enough training and is competent to practise safely. Certificates of attendance provide verifiable CPD which is logged and quantified.
2. Quality improvement activity—doctors are expected to be engaged in quality improvement activities such as audits and feasibility studies. This should be shown at each revalidation cycle whilst the appraisal process ensures that this is done within a given 5-year cycle
3. Significant events (any incident which could have resulted in serious harm to patients)—these events should be logged and documented and discussed at the yearly appraisal. This review process leads to lessons learnt and dissipated to prevent similar events from happening again.
4. Feedback from colleagues—15 feedback forms (usually online) is the recommendation for every revalidation cycle.
5. Feedback from patients—10–20 completed and returned feedback forms (usually online) is recommended for every revalidation cycle.
6. Review of complaints and compliments—any complaints and/or compliments should be documented. These complaints and compliments form part of the appraisal process.

How often does revalidation take place?

Each medical practitioner should undertake revalidation for the GMC every 5 years.

When should all the documentation be submitted?

Each doctor is notified of the revalidation date 6 months in advance and is invited by the GMC to confirm his/her details online. The doctor is then given formal notice 4 months prior to the revalidation date—this is known as the statutory notice period.

The Responsible Officer submits the recommendation on or before the validation date and the GMC makes the final decision based on the recommendation.

At each revalidation cycle, the following need to be produced:

- Personal details (including your GMC reference number).
- Job plan schedule.
- Collation of annual appraisal documentation.
- Personal development plans and their review.
- Probity, based on the MSF and previous performance.

What is the difference between revalidation for a qualified doctor and a trainee?

The designated body responsible for revalidation of a qualified doctor is the GMC, whereas for a trainee it is regional Local Education Training Boards. LETBs are local committees for Health Education England (HEE). The LETB will make a recommendation to revalidate a trainee following the yearly ARCP (Annual Review of Competence Progression) process.

Medical doctors in training include the following:

- newly qualified doctors, foundation year doctors (FY)
- doctors in an approved training programme or post
- doctors in a fixed training programme—known as a fixed term specialty training programme (FTSTP)
- those in a locum position for training—locum appointment for training (LAT).

What are the possible outcomes from the revalidation process?

The result of the revalidation process takes 4–6 weeks to be released. If the requirements were met but the information submitted was incomplete, two possible outcomes arise:

- request for the missing information
- initiation of licence withdrawal

If the requirements were not met, the possible outcomes include the following:

- re-sit the revalidation process
- provide the missing information that could validate the process
- resubmit the deficient assessment forming part of the portfolio reflecting the cause for failing to pass the revalidation assessment
- relinquish licence/have licence revoked
- undergo a fitness to practise committee investigation

## Further Readings

BMA (2008) SASC implementation guidance – programmed activities. https://www.bma.org.uk/-/media/files/pdfs/practical%20advice%20at%20work/job%20planning/sascpadossier1208.pdf?la=en. Accessed Jan 2020

GMC (2013) Good medical practice – guidance. https://www.gmc-uk.org/-/media/documents/Good_medical_practice___English_1215.pdf_51527435.pdf. Accessed Jan 2019

NHS England (2020a) Our NHS People Promise. https://www.england.nhs.uk/wp-content/uploads/2020/07/Our_NHS_People_Promise.pdf. Accessed Jan 2021

NHS England (2020b) We are the NHS: people plan for 2020/2021 - action for us all. https://www.england.nhs.uk/wp-content/uploads/2020/07/We_Are_The_NHS_Action_For_All_Of_Us_FINAL_24_08_20.pdf. Accessed Jan 2021

NHS Revalidation Support Team (2014a) Medical appraisal guide - a guide to medical appraisal for revalidation in England. https://www.england.nhs.uk/revalidation/wp-content/uploads/sites/10/2014/02/rst-medical-app-guide-2013.pdf. Accessed Jan 2019

NHS Revalidation Support Team (2014b) Early benefits an impact of medical revalidation: report on research findings in year one. https://www.england.nhs.uk/revalidation/wp-content/uploads/sites/10/2014/03/earl-ben-impact-mr-report.pdf. Accessed Jan 2019

The King's Fund (2014) Medical revalidation from compliance to commitment. https://www.kingsfund.org.uk/sites/default/files/field/field_publication_file/medical-validation-vijaya-nath-mar14.pdf. Accessed Jan 2019

# Ethical Practice and Medico-legal Themes in the NHS

# 6

## 6.1 Introduction

Ethics govern our behaviour and attitude to both colleagues and patients on a daily basis. In the UK, a set of obligations and regulations, outlined in the Medical Act 1983, are enforced by the GMC and the GDC. To maintain the high standards of the medical and dental professions, these regulations should be adhered to. It is essential to show dignity and respect to all patients at all times.

Legislation is in place to protect patient confidentiality, namely, Data Protection Act 1998, Access to Health Records Act 1990, Human Rights Act 1998, Computer Misuse Act 1990, and NHS Act 2006. However, health professionals may on occasion be required by law to disclose certain information, regardless of patient consent, but should also ensure that they do not disclose more information than is necessary. Where such a statutory requirement exists, patient consent to disclosure is not necessary. Patients have no right to refuse but they should be generally aware of the disclosure and that it is to a secure authority. Examples of statutory disclosures include: Public Health (Control of Disease) Act 1984, Abortion Regulations 1991, Reporting of Injuries, Disease and Dangerous Occurrences Regulation 1985, Road Traffic Act 1998, Terrorism Act 2000, and The Information Sharing Index Regulations (England) 2007. Disclosures can also be required by the police, solicitors, courts, tribunals and regulatory bodies.

## 6.2 Ethics in Everyday Practice

There are four core principles in medical ethics: autonomy, beneficence, non-maleficence and justice.

**Autonomy**

This refers to the patient's total freedom to accept or refuse to undertake a specific procedure based on the perceived risks and benefits.



S. Abela, *Leadership and Management in Healthcare*,
https://doi.org/10.1007/978-3-031-21025-9_6

Clinical example in daily practice: a patient who is a Jehovah's Witness attends his GP practice requesting surgery to repair a cleft palate. This usually entails a bone graft taken from the hip, but the refusal of the patient to accept a blood transfusion if needed, increases the complexity of any surgical consequences.

**Beneficence**

This refers to the requirement of doctors to promote the course of action that they believe is in the best interests of the patient.

Clinical example in daily practice: An FY1 doctor examines a patient presenting with a urological problem, the doctor's area of interest. The young doctor is faced with an interesting and challenging problem and becomes excited about managing it himself; however, he goes out of his way to approach a more senior member of staff who is better qualified to deal with the matter.

**Non-maleficence**

This refers to the duty a doctor has to do no harm or allow harm to be caused to a patient through neglect.

Clinical example in daily practice: A female patient attends a routine gynaecological appointment and is given two options: to accept that the benign lump in her breast was an incidental finding and can be ignored, or consent to a mastectomy with all the possible attendant complications. The second option should not be considered given the risks to which the patient will be exposed, completely outweighing the benefits.

**Justice**

This requires doctors to consider whether an action is ethical or otherwise, and also whether it is compatible with the law and the rights of the individual, and whether it is fair and balanced from society's perspective.

Clinical example in daily practice: A GP has a full list of patients booked for his surgery and just one emergency slot available. In the morning two patients phone the practice requesting an emergency appointment: a 15-year-old boy who has just noticed a suspicious lesion on his back which is hard and has a family history of melanoma and a 70-year-old woman who has a persistent headache that has not responded to paracetamol. The GP should not favour the younger patient based on the younger age as this would be unjust and unfair towards the older patient. However, the GP should favour the younger patient based on the clinical priority.

Other values that a medical clinician should demonstrate include:

- Respect and dignity
- Truthfulness and honesty

## 6.3 Confidentiality and Consent

Confidentiality is an essential requirement for the preservation of trust between patients and health professionals and is subject to legal and ethical safeguards. Patient information should be requested by the treating practitioner and held centrally and securely within the institution's hardware unless there is a compelling reason why not.

All patient information which can be in written, digital, photographic or audio form should be kept confidential to avoid identifying the patient.

There are two main types of consent:

- *Expressed consent*: A patient is offered an investigation or treatment and agrees to that treatment; this consent can be given in verbal or written form.
- *Implied consent*: This occurs when the patient adopts particular behaviours consistent with demonstrating that they have understood the doctor's request by complying with the request, such as when a patient extends their arm to have their blood pressure monitored.

### 6.3.1 Consent to Release Information

Patients must be asked for permission before releasing any identifiable information.

Clinical example in daily practice: A chest X-ray requested for a patient with acute asthma and cardiomyopathy forms part of the information needed to complete a case report for a journal article. In such an instance the clinician should obtain written permission from the patient and any identifying features in the material should be rendered anonymous in the publication.

Patient consent can either be verbal or written and explicit or implied.

Clinical example in daily practice: A patient attends a dermatology appointment and allows an examination of a suspect naevus, followed by a biopsy procedure. Although no written consent was obtained, implied consent was granted simply by allowing the examination to take place.

Consent for treatment can be withdrawn at any stage by the patient and the health professional should take the necessary steps to halt the progress or stop any treatment procedures in place pertaining to a patient.

Clinical example in daily practice: A patient who gave written consent at the start of a clinical trial to have all his participation data published, withdraws his consent 1 month after the trial starts. All of the trial data relating to that patient will be rendered non-publishable. If the patient decides to withdraw from the study completely, he would then be classified as a drop-out in the investigation.

### 6.3.2 Authority to Access Confidential Information

Information can be shared between treating clinicians or other health professionals directly involved in a patient's care on a 'need to know basis'. But in the case of multi-agency involvement, the patient's consent should be sought beforehand unless there is public interest or if required by law.

## 6.4 Consent for Treatment

Obtaining consent from patients before a procedure forms the basis of everyday medical practice. Obtaining consent must be voluntarily, an informed decision and with no compromises on the patients' decision-making capabilities.

### 6.4.1 Patient's Consent to Treatment

The consenting procedure is evidence of a patient's self-determination in accepting a particular intervention to assess/manage their condition. There should be complete freedom on the part of the individual.

The medical professional should in no way interfere or impose the intervention onto the patient and the patient has the right to withdraw this consent at any stage during treatment.

The capability of a patient to make his or her own decision must also be assessed. Capacity can be impaired in case of mental illness, or due to unconsciousness, or the influence of drugs including alcohol. Mental capacity should be assessed if doubts exist; however, a doctor should always act in the patient's best interests.

Although the consenting of patients is not a legal obligation, it is a highly recommended process that should be undertaken prior to starting any form of treatment. The ideal consenting procedure involves the following:

- a full explanation of the procedure and/or investigation
- the reasons why the specific procedure is required
- other possible options/alternatives
- the consequences if this procedure/investigation is not carried out
- the pros and cons of carrying out this procedure/investigation
- a breakdown of all costs involved if treatment is being carried out in a non-NHS organisation
- all the risks and benefits for each treatment option

All patients above the age of 16 years can consent. If the patient is younger, Fraser's principles for competency (formerly known as Gillick competency) would apply, but ideally consent would also be obtained from the patient's guardians.

Most trusts recognise four types of consent forms designed to meet the needs of different groups of patients at different times; however, these might vary from one trust to another:

- Consent form 1: for patients able to consent for themselves.
- Consent form 2: for those with parental responsibility, consenting on behalf of a child/young person.
- Consent form 3: for patients able to consent for themselves and for those with parental responsibility consenting on behalf of a child/young person, where the procedure does not involve any impairment of consciousness (the patient is expected to remain alert during the procedure). This is usually used in elective cases, but the use of this form is optional as consent form type 1 and 2 can also apply
- Consent form 4: for adults who lack capacity to consent to a particular treatment. Treatment has to be in their 'best interests'. This form requires health professionals to document both how the procedure will benefit the patient and the reasons for proceeding. It also allows the involvement of those close to the patient in making this healthcare decision to be documented.

In the case of minors, when it is felt that parents or guardians are not making the best decision for their child, a trust or a medical professional can take a case to court for the final decision to be taken by a tribunal.

### 6.4.2 Consent for the Use of Human Tissue

Use of biopsies and human tissue for scientific purposes should be in line with The Human Tissue Act 2004.

The Act demands that the patient's consent is obtained for:

- storage, research, transplantation or post-mortem examination purposes following biopsies of a patient's organ(s) or tissue
- storage, research, transplantation or post-mortem examination purposes of a deceased patient's organ or biopsy

### 6.4.3 Consent for Clinical Photography/Video Recordings

Clinical photography and/or video recordings form part of the patients' records. Written consent for this type of record should also be obtained. There are three levels of consent and each trust will have its own consent forms:

- photographs/video recordings to be stored in the patient's health records
- photographs/video recordings to be placed in the patient's health records and for educational purposes

- photographs/video recordings to be placed in the patient's health records, for educational purposes and for publication and/or research.

### 6.4.4 Consent for Fertility Treatments

The Human Fertilisation and Embryology Act 1990 (as amended by the Human Fertilisation and Embryology Act 2008) acts as a legal framework across the UK for all those involved in fertility treatments. It defines the rights of all the parties involved in fertility treatments including donors, patients and the children who may be involved in the treatment.

The Act also restricts research on human embryos for specific purposes and places time limits on the storage of embryos, eggs and sperm. The Human Fertilisation and Embryology Authority (HFEA) is the regulator for fertility clinics. The HFEA was created under the Act to regulate the licencing and compliance of treatment clinics and research centres and monitor unethical fertilisation methods and unethical destruction of fertilised embryos.

In fertility treatments, similar to other medical treatments, seeking the patients' consent should pre-empt any other intervention. Consent is important in these types of treatments due to the very serious legal implications of who is recognised as the parent/guardian of the offspring.

Consent is not only related to usage of the eggs and/or sperm but also to storage long term and the number of gametes or blastocyst embryos stored and permitted to be transferred via In Vitro Fertilisation (IVF).

Consent in such circumstances will therefore certainly involve: storage duration, type of treatment, breakdown of fees if performed in a non-NHS organisation, parental responsibility and use of personal information.

## 6.5 Reporting: Duty of Candour

In a post-Francis era, the duty of candour is an obligation and the 'whistleblowing' policy is very closely intertwined with this moral obligation. Following the mid-Staffordshire investigations, 290 recommendations were listed, one of which involved raising concerns about colleagues. In general, once suspicions are raised and verified:

- raise concerns with the colleague directly in an informal manner if this is appropriate.
- put the patients' interest and safety first.
- manage the problem directly.
- report your concerns to your colleague's line manager.
- take further advice if needed by managerial staff or external sources once all local measures have been exhausted.

## 6.6 Proof of Negligence

In a court of law there is a four-fold test for proof negligence.

1. The first stage is to prove 'duty of care' where a person is directly involved or has undertaken activities that might directly harm another person.
2. The second stage is determining that the duty of care has been breached. This is confirmed by applying the 'Bolam test'. This principle has become the gold standard on which a judgement against a health professional is made; a judge in a court of law assesses the doctor's decision against the consensus of a group of doctors with similar expertise to the doctor against whom the claim is being made. The 'Bolam test' can be applied in addition to the 'Montgomery test', also known as the 'test of materiality'. The Montgomery test does not test the degree of reasonable decision-making, but instead assesses the relaying of significance of risk to a patient if they decide to go ahead with the procedure.
3. The third stage is to determine the causal association between the action and/or decision-making by the doctor and the effects on the patient.
4. The fourth stage is to determine the nature and extent of the damages arisen as a result of the act of negligence experienced.

## Further Readings

General Medical Council (2008) Consent: patients and doctors making decisions together – guidance. https://www.gmc-uk.org/static/documents/content/Consent_-_English_0617.pdf. Accessed Jan 2020

General Medical Council (2009) Confidentiality – guidance. https://www.gmc-uk.org/-/media/documents/Confidentiality_good_practice_in_handling_patient_information___English_0417.pdf_70080105.pdf. Accessed Jan 2020

General Medical Council (2010) Good practice in research and consent to research – guidance. www.gmc-uk.org/static/documents/content/Good_practice_in_research_and_consent_to_research.pdf. Accessed Dec 2019

General Medical Council (2012) Raising and acting on concerns about patient safety – guidance. www.gmc-uk.org/static/documents/content/Raising_and_acting_on_concerns_about_patient_safety_-_English_1015.pdf. Accessed Dec 2019

General Medical Council (2013) Financial and commercial arrangements and conflicts of interest – guidance. www.gmc-uk.org/static/documents/content/Financial_and_commercial_arrangements_and_conflicts_of_interest.pdf. Accessed Dec 2019

Gillon R (1994) Medical ethics: four principles plus attention to scope. BMJ 309:184

Human Fertilisation and Embryology Act 1990 (n.d.). http://www.legislation.gov.uk/ukpga/1990/37/pdfs/ukpga_19900037_en.pdf. Accessed Dec 2019

Human Fertilisation and Embryology Act 2008 (n.d.). http://www.legislation.gov.uk/ukpga/2008/22/pdfs/ukpga_20080022_en.pdf. Accessed Dec 2019

Human Tissue Act 2004 (n.d.). www.legislation.gov.uk/ukpga/2004/30/pdfs/ukpga_20040030_en.pdf. Accessed Dec 2018

Mental Capacity Act 2005 (n.d.). http://www.legislation.gov.uk/ukpga/2005/9/pdfs/ukpga_20050009_en.pdf. Accessed Dec 2019

# 7 Clinical Effectiveness and Clinical Audit

## 7.1 Introduction

Modern medicine requires that clinical effectiveness is at the core of daily medical practice. Clinical governance is key for this to be established routinely by making patient-centred decisions and orientate service to focus solely on the individual patients.

## 7.2 Clinical Effectiveness

The Department of Health (DH) defines clinical effectiveness as: 'the application of the best knowledge, derived from research, clinical experience and patient preferences to achieve optimum processes and outcomes of care for patients. The process involves a framework of informing, changing and monitoring practice'.

Clinical effectiveness is one of the key pillars of clinical governance and, together with regular clinical audits and high quality research, excellence in healthcare can readily be achieved. Clinical effectiveness aims to use evidence-based medicine to ensure the best possible outcomes post-operatively and make health provision cost-effective. The DH defines clinical effectiveness as the '5 rights': 'doing the right thing, the right way, at the right time, at the right place, with the right outcome'.

Clinical effectiveness is an umbrella term for the overall quality of care given to patients. Each trust will have several specialised groups and committees to collaborate and interlink their activities to develop this strategy and implement the necessary changes: These include the following:

- Clinical Governance Committee
- Clinical Effectiveness and Research Group
- Complaints Team
- Confidentiality and Caldicott Guardian



S. Abela, *Leadership and Management in Healthcare*,
https://doi.org/10.1007/978-3-031-21025-9_7

- Clinical Risk Management Team
- Educational Supervisors and Responsible Officers
- Audit and Research Committee

### 7.2.1 The Stages of Clinical Effectiveness

Achieving clinical effectiveness involves a cycle of three stages which have to be continually adopted (Fig. 7.1):

- Stage 1: obtaining information/evidence—All doctors should be aware of the latest evidence available in the literature, and should be able to demonstrate this in the appraisals.
- Stage 2: implementing change—Medical practice should be based on the latest evidence available, and evidence-based medicine should form the core of all decision-making processes.

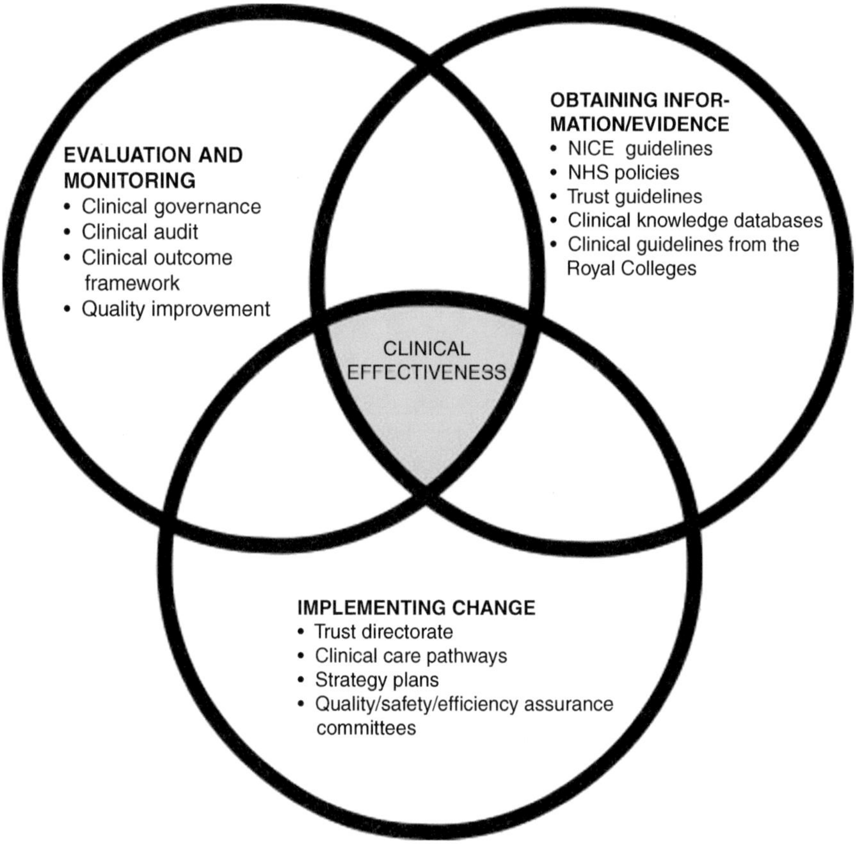


**Fig. 7.1** The three stages of clinical effectiveness

- Stage 3: evaluation and monitoring—An assessment of the impact of new practice based on evidence should be obtained through audits, measuring outcomes and obtaining patient questionnaires and feedback.

## 7.3 Clinical Governance

This is a term introduced in 1998 by Scally and Donaldson which can be defined as 'a framework through which NHS organisations are accountable for continually improving the quality of their services and safeguarding high standards of care by creating an environment in which excellence in clinical care will flourish'. It is based on 7 pillars:

- clinical effectiveness
- risk management effectiveness
- patient experience
- communication effectiveness
- resource effectiveness
- strategic effectiveness
- learning effectiveness

### 7.3.1 Research Governance

Similar to clinical governance, research governance is the adherence to the principles of safe and effective research. The Research Governance Framework (RGF) in 2005 defined a set of rules and regulations to ensure safe research practices. In 2015, the RGF became a non-departmental public body (NDPB) and has now been superseded by the Health Research Authority (HRA).

**The Health Research Authority**

The HRA's principles are based on the Care Act (2014). The HRA aims to protect the public from health and social care research. This protection ensures that the public benefits from ethically approved research and has transparent results delivered. It also oversees research committees and organisations to ensure a safe framework and promotes readily available information such as patient information sheets and consent forms detailing the risks and benefits in research trials.

The HRA creates a single framework for all the research activity carried out in the UK, enabling relaying of all research findings to the public for better use. It has three main committees and provides an integrated service.

Research Ethics Committee: The REC is made up of professionals and lay people and it oversees applications and passes judgements about the ethical nature of research projects. The processing of research applications by the REC ensures monitoring of:

- the patient's rights
- the patient's dignity
- the patient's safety

The Declaration of Helsinki 2008 states that, first and foremost, no harm should occur to the patient as a result of a research study and that any new product or intervention is safe for all patients.

Gene Therapy Advisory Committee: The GTAC processes applications for any clinical trials involving gene therapy.

Confidentiality Advisory Group: The CAG protects and ensures appropriate use of confidential patient information during and after the research project.

The HRA's ultimate mandate is to regulate and streamline research projects by approving or declining all submitted healthcare research project applications, thus allowing local NHS providers to concentrate on the research delivery.

Researchers must also adhere to the Clinical Trial Regulations 2004 which defined the roles of the chief and principal investigators in a research project. The chief investigator is the person with the overall responsibility for running the study, whilst the principal investigator is the person carrying out the research.

Medicines and Healthcare Products Regulatory Agency: The MHRA is an executive agency sponsored by the Department of Health and Social Care (DHSC).

This agency regulating the safe use of medicines and medical devices despite the similar abbreviation, should not be confused with HRA.

This agency ensures:

- standards of safety, quality and efficacy in medicines, medical devices and blood components for transfusion
- secure safe supply chains for medicines, medical devices and blood components
- promotion of international standardisation of safety for biological medicines
- the education of the public and healthcare professionals about the risks and effective use of medicines, medical devices and blood components
- the support of innovation and research and development that is beneficial to public health
- influence on national and international regulatory frameworks to protecting pub lic health

The MHRA's priorities have been comprehensively listed in the 5-year Corporate Plan (2018–2023).

### 7.3.2 Non-NHS Research Projects

HRA approval processes apply to project-based research taking place in NHS organisations and NHS-contracted primary care services. HRA approval does not cover non-NHS organisations or institutions that are seeking to deliver research projects. Non-NHS Site-Specific Information (SSI) forms should be sent to the Research Ethics Committee (REC).

Studies which are being undertaken by independent healthcare providers may still need to be assessed for ethical approval from an NHS REC. Such trials include the investigations of interventional medical products (IMPs), investigations that involve patients who are unable to consent: in England approval for these individuals falls under the Mental Capacity Act and in Scotland approval falls under the Adults with Incapacity Act. For research projects involving human tissue, approval is set out in the Governance Arrangements for Research Ethics Committees (GAfREC).

## 7.4 Clinical Audit

Clinical audit is defined as 'a quality improvement process that seeks to improve patient care and outcomes through systematic review of care against explicit criteria and the implementation of change'. Every clinical audit must be registered at the Research and Audit Department of each hospital trust and a registration number obtained.

### 7.4.1 Classification of Clinical Audits

Several types of classification have been used based on timing, geographical spread of the audit being undertaken and the type of the audit.

Classification based on timing:

- prospective or
- retrospective, following a reported clinical incident which the investigation officer is commissioned to assess

Classification based on geographical spread of the audit:

- local
- regional
- national

Classification based on audit type:

- clinic-based
- laboratory-based
- radiography-based
- risk management

### 7.4.2 The Clinical Audit Cycle

Clinical audit is a quality control process which follows a cyclical pattern (Fig. 7.2).

- The process is initiated by observing a problem or deficiency in the service provision.
- Criteria (ideal standards and targets) are then set against which the service should be evaluated.

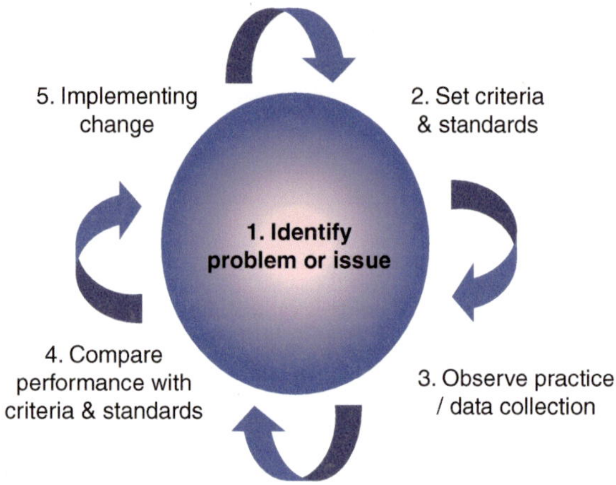


**Fig. 7.2** The clinical audit cycle. This figure is reproduced from Wikipedia under the CC BY-SA 3.0 licence

- Data on current practice is collected and reviewed.
- Performance is then compared to the previously set standards and criteria.
- The cycle ends by implementing the changes required.

As a minimum, each audit process requires at least two of these cycles: the first to review practice, and recommend and implement changes, and a second to review the impact of the changes and recommend further changes if necessary. Some audit cycles are ongoing and so go round this cycle continuously.

### 7.4.3 Advantages of Clinical Audit

A clinical audit is a mechanism to establish if the healthcare currently provided is in line with the standards set. It is an improvement-seeking tool which allows care providers and patients know where their service is doing well and where there are specific deficiencies.

Clinical audits are usually inexpensive and cost-effective and can be carried out by clinicians without the need of additional administrative staff. They can be carried out over a specific timeframe and results are obtained without the need for complex statistical analysis.

### 7.4.4 Difference Between Clinical Audit and Clinical Research

A clinical audit is usually part of a cyclical process where the main aim is to assess the current method of healthcare provision; it is a quality-control exercise that assesses the need for improvement and, following changes, checks again to confirm an improvement. Clinical research, on the other hand, aims to improve understanding by providing new evidence following strict adherence to the research protocol. The main differences are shown in Table 7.1.

**Table 7.1** Comparison of clinical audit with clinical research

| Clinical audit | Clinical research |
|---|---|
| Designed to produce information about the quality of care provided | Designed to generate new knowledge about medical practice |
| Designed to assess success against targets | Designed to test a null hypothesis; in the case of qualitative studies, a trend or feedback is usually obtained from existing methodologies |
| Outcomes are measured against a set standard | Addresses defined aims and objectives and should be replicable by other research teams |
| Leads to improvement in the delivery of care by implementing changes to the service | May involve evaluating and comparing different interventions with one acting as a control or benchmark; in qualitative research, feedback on patient experience is obtained via validated tools |
| Does not require complex statistical analysis | Requires specialist statistics |
| Does not require an ethical approval process | Ethical approval is always required |
| Does not involve provision of new treatments | May involve new medicinal products or new devices |

### 7.4.5 National Clinical Audits

National clinical audits, as the name implies, are carried out at a national level in contrast to local audits which are typically carried out in a local NHS institution.

**The National Clinical Audit and Patient Outcomes Programme**

See: www.hqip.org.uk/national-programmes/a-z-of-nca

The National Clinical Audit and Patient Outcomes Programme (NCAPOP) is commissioned on behalf of NHS England by the HQIP (see Sect. 2.2.5). The programme comprises over 30 national audits related to some of the most commonly occurring medical conditions. Local clinicians provide the data which collectively produces a national standard and outcomes for each condition. NCAPOP provides outcomes for the individual local trusts which can also be benchmarked against national standards.

An example is the Sentinel Stroke National Audit Programme (SSNAP) which aims to improve the quality of stroke care by auditing local stroke services against the national standards, which are also part of NICE quality standards (see Sect. 1.2.5).

A secondary aim of NCAPOP is to provide the Clinical Outcome Review Programme (CORP) with reports on adverse effects to reduce negative outcomes.

**National Quality Improvement and Clinical Audit Network**

See: www.nqican.org.uk

The National Quality Improvement and Clinical Audit Network (NQICAN) brings together the 15 regional clinical audit/effectiveness networks in England and works closely with NHS England, NICE and HQIP. The aim of NQICAN is to support staff working in health and social care organisations in these areas, providing them with training, resources and raising any concerns at a national level.

**National Advisory Group on Clinical Audit and Enquiries**

See: https://www.gov.uk/government/groups/national-advisory-group-on-clinical-audit-and-enquiries

The National Advisory Group on Clinical Audit and Enquiries NCAAG provides policy and strategic advice to NHS England on clinical audit and enquiries, with the aim of:

- enhancing the existing programme of national clinical audits
- supporting the many NHS staff involved in local audits and enquiries in their own trusts
- seeking to improve connections, such as results from different national clinical audits

## 7.5 Achieving Clinical Effectiveness

Clinical audit on its own will not achieve clinical excellence or clinical effectiveness. So, each trust sets up an Effectiveness Group to develop an Effectiveness Strategy, which incorporates:

- NICE guidelines and evidence-based practice
- mortality, morbidity and survival reviews
- research and service evaluation
- education and training of staff
- quality forums
- continuous updating of policies
- monitoring and improving outcomes
- financial control by Monitor (now part of NHS Improvement)

Every trust issues a vision and strategy to improve clinical effectiveness. This strategy can change year on year depending on the targets that need to be achieved.

Table 7.2 systematically lists the objective needed to implement clinical effectiveness within a typical UK hospital. It also lists the responsible officer, the group and the board level at which the responsible officer operates within the hospital hierarchy.

**Table 7.2** Responsibility and monitoring of clinical effectiveness

| Objective | Responsible person | Monitoring and implementation group | Group's position in the hospital structure |
|---|---|---|---|
| Practice audit | Audit manager | Audit and Research Committee | Sub-committee to the board of directors |
| NICE and national guidelines | Effectiveness coordinator | Clinical Governance Committee | Committee with a direct link to the board of directors |
| Evidence-based practice | Audit and research officers | Clinical Effectiveness Group | Part of the operational and performance sub-committee; this is directly linked to the operational board and their duties are linked to the trust executive committee |
| Mortality reviews | Medical director | Patient Safety Committee | Part of the assurance, risk and quality sub-committee; this is directly linked to the quality assurance committee, which responds to the governance committee |
| Research and service evaluation | Audit and research manager | Audit and Research Committee | The audit and research sub-committee is directly linked to the board of directors |
| Quality of treatment | Medical director | Patient Safety Committee | This sub-committee is directly linked to the governance committee which in turn is linked to the board of directors |
| Policies and procedures | Clinical effectiveness facilitators | Clinical Governance Committee | Part of the operational and performance sub-committee which is in turn linked to the operational board |
| Quality and assurance | Risk manager | Executive Management Team | A sub-committee to the board of directors |

## Further Readings

Care Act (2014). www.legislation.gov.uk/ukpga/2014/23/pdfs/ukpga_20140023_en.pdf. Accessed Dec 2019

Healthcare Quality Improvement Partnership (2011) Guide to using quality improvement tools to drive clinical audits – guidance. www.hqip.org.uk/public/cms/253/625/19/193/HQIP-Guide-to-Using-Quality-Improvement-Tools-to-Drive-CA-2011.pdf?realName=NIgOW4.pdf&v=0. Accessed Dec 2018

Health Research Authority (2014) HRA and research sponsor responsibilities – consultation. https://www.hra.nhs.uk/documents/796/sponsors-responsibilities-consultation-paper.pdf. Accessed Dec 2019

MHRA (2013) Documents outlining the Medicines & Healthcare products Regulatory Agency's strategic direction for 2013–18 including our mission, aims and objectives for this five year period—corporate report. www.gov.uk/government/publications/mhra-corporate-plan-2013-to-2018. Accessed Dec 2019

MHRA (2016) An update of the Medicines & Healthcare products Regulatory Agency's 2013–18 Corporate Plan. https://assets.publishing.service.gov.uk/government/uploads/system/uploads/attachment_data/file/519539/Medicines_and_Healthcare_products_Regulatory_Agency_Corporate_Plan_Refresh_2016.pdf. Accessed Dec 2019

Southport and Ormskirk Hospital NHS Trust (2013) Quality and governance business unit – clinical effectiveness strategy. www.southportandormskirk.nhs.uk/pdfs/Clinical-Effectiveness-Strategy.pdf. Accessed Dec 2019

# Trainee Performance and Assessment in the NHS

# 8

## 8.1 Introduction

Medical and dental training in the UK is regulated by the GMC and the GDC. Before addressing the appraisal and assessment processes, it is important first to understand the structure which underpins the delivery, regulation and monitoring of education and training within the NHS.

## 8.2 The Structure

This refers to the bodies, organisations and institutions involved in the running and regulation of training for all healthcare professionals.

### 8.2.1 The Regulators

The GMC and the GDC are the two main regulators in the UK.

**The General Medical Council**

See: www.gmc-uk.org

The GMC was established in the Medical Act 1858. This independent organisation has two major roles: to protect patients and to improve medical education and practice across the UK. It sets standards for doctors, oversees their training and education, manages the UK medical register, investigates and acts on concerns from patients and maintains standards through revalidation. Further information can be found in Sect. 4.3.3.



S. Abela, *Leadership and Management in Healthcare*,
https://doi.org/10.1007/978-3-031-21025-9_8

**The General Dental Council**

See: www.gdc-uk.org

The GDC was established in 1956 by an amendment to the Dentist Act 1948. It registers all qualified dentists and other dental healthcare professionals. It sets standards for dental education and regulates the dental and dental care professions. Further information can be found in Sect. 4.3.2.

### 8.2.2 Postgraduate Training Bodies

Training for doctors and dentists is set and monitored by the professional colleges. The colleges set standards for training through the development of the curriculum, summative examinations (college examinations) and formative assessments. These formative assessments, which include work-based assessments, are collected as evidence of training in the E-portfolio. The colleges awards CCT (certificate of completion of training) to successful candidates.

**NHS Deaneries and Local Education and Training Boards**

See: https://hee.nhs.uk

An NHS deanery is a regional organisation responsible for postgraduate medical and dental training within the NHS to standards set by the GMC and GDC. Restructuring of NHS England in 2013 led to deaneries being incorporated into new bodies known as local education and training boards (LETBs). The deanery is responsible for coordinating postgraduate medical and dental education within a region to standards set by the GMC and the GDC. Deaneries are advised by specialist training committees (STCs).

STCs are made up of a chair, a training programme director/s (TPD), head of school of medicine, a trainee representative, an associate dean, a deanery workforce representative and a training representative from the respective trusts. The role of the STCs is to ensure that the highest levels of training are being achieved in each specialty. The adherence to the Gold Guide is key, a reference guide for postgraduate Specialty Training in the UK.

In the NHS reforms of April 2013, 13 regional LETBs were set up. They are statutory committees of HEE with three major functions: to identify and agree the local needs for education and training, to plan and commission high quality education and training in the region, and to support national workforce priorities set by Health Education England (HEE).

**NHS Training Leadership and Oversight**

Health Education England

See: https://hee.nhs.uk

HEE was originally established as a Special Health Authority (SpHA) in 2012. Since 2015, it is a non-departmental public body under the provisions of the Care Act 2014.

The role of HEE is to provide leadership for the new education and training system. It ensures that the shape and skills of the future health and public health workforce evolve to maintain high quality outcomes for patients in the face of demographic and technological change. It supports healthcare providers and clinicians to allow them to take greater responsibility for planning and commissioning education and training through the development of LETBs.

The establishment and development of HEE was set out in 'Liberating the NHS: Developing the Healthcare Workforce, From Design to Delivery', the Government's policy for a new system for planning the commissioning of education and training.

The key national functions of HEE include:

- Providing national leadership for planning and developing the whole healthcare and public health workforce.
- Authorising and supporting development of LETBs and holding them to account.
- Promoting high quality education and training which is responsive to the changing needs of patients and communities and delivered to standards set by regulators.
- Allocating and accounting for NHS education and training resources—ensuring transparency, fairness and efficiency in investments made across England.
- Ensuring security of supply of a professionally qualified clinical workforce.
- Assisting the spread of innovation across the NHS in order to improve quality of care.
- Delivering against the national Education Outcomes Framework to ensure the allocation of education and training resources is linked to quantifiable improvements.

The HEE works with the Allied Health Professions advisory board, the Nursing and Midwifery professional advisory board and Medical Education England's programme boards for dentistry, healthcare science, medical and pharmacy and public health.

**Postgraduate Schools**

Within individual LETBs, postgraduate schools provide individualised faculty training for each trainee. The training consists of three main components:

1. The core training component—The trainee is provided with the skills and knowledge necessary to meet the expected standards of a trainee within the respective specialty. Clinically, the trainee is continuously supervised by the clinical supervisor. The clinical supervisor reports the rate of progress of the individual trainee to the educational supervisor who in turn relays the information to the training programme director. The latter ultimately reports progress to the Postgraduate Dean at the regional LETB.
2. A system of support and professional development—The trainee is provided with support throughout his/her training period to ensure a successful training pathway. Throughout the duration of the training, support for the trainee is also available from, for example, Occupational Health, HumanResources, and councillors provided by the department or LETB.

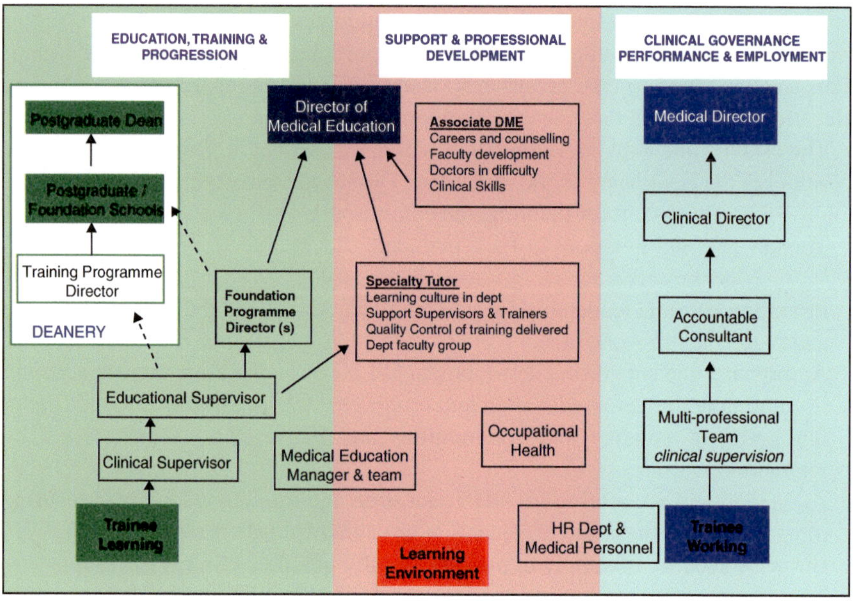


**Fig. 8.1** The structure of governance within the medical training process, courtesy of NACT UK, on behalf of the Quality Management Subgroup of JACSTAG 2008

3. A structure that enables employment and performance assessment—The trainee will always be provided with feedback from colleagues, supervising Consultants, the Clinical Director and the Medical Director, with the latter being the responsible officer for clinicians within a hospital structure.

Figure 8.1 illustrates the structure for postgraduate education and training and the components described above. This process underpins assessments and the annual review of competence progression until the CCT stage.

## 8.3 The Process

Understanding the structure shown in Fig. 8.1 helps understanding of the process that underpins trainee and senior staff appraisal, performance assessment and peer review. This is best divided into pre-CCT and post-CCT.

The pre-CCT is the phase of training leading to, as the name implies, a certificate of completion of training.

The post-CCT is the abbreviation for post completion of certificate training and aims to deliver higher training enabling the trainee to achieve abilities to manage the most complex of medical problems associated with the respective specialty. Within the medical field, this is referred to as sub-specialty or super-specialty training. This qualification deemed to be akin to a fellowship entitles the trainee to apply for very senior positions within an NHS trust such as a consultant post.

### 8.3.1 Pre-CCT Appraisal

The pre-CCT appraisal is an educational evaluation to identify a trainee's development needs, provide feedback on their performance and record progress. Appraisal meetings are usually held with an educational supervisor at the start, middle and end of each year and with clinical supervisors for each post.

**Annual Review of Competence Progression**

See: https://www.hee.nhs.uk/our-work/annual-review-competency-progression

ARCP is an evidence-based panel review of a trainee's progress. The panel reports the outcome of this review to the Training Programme Director (TPD), the trainee and the trainee's employers. Further details of the ARCP process for foundation doctors can be found on the website.

Personnel involved in the ARCP process.

Several professionals are involved in the training pathway of medical and dental trainees. Their individual positions and roles in the ARCP are set out below.

*Clinical Supervisor*: a trainer who is selected and appropriately trained to be responsible for overseeing a trainee's clinical work and providing constructive feedback during a training placement. Clinical supervisors provide induction and end of module appraisal and they usually conduct workplace-based assessments (WPBA) for the period of modular training.

*Educational Supervisor*: a trainer who is selected to be responsible for the overall supervision and management of a trainee's educational progress during a training placement or series of placements for a minimum of 1 year. The Educational Supervisor conducts induction, mid-term and end of year appraisals and provides a structured report to inform the ARCP process.

*Training Programme Director*: a senior clinician appointed by the deanery and postgraduate school to oversee the management of the specialty training programme.

*Head of School*: senior consultant within the deanery who provides strategic leadership for the development of the postgraduate school. The school provides and co-ordinates the education and training of doctors or dentists within the specialty.

*Regional Advisor*: represents the views of the college in relevant matters within their regions. They work closely with Postgraduate Deans, serve on the relevant local committees, and advise the President or Council on aspects of training and clinical standards within their local regions. Regional Advisors may also sit on other college committees.

*College Tutor*: co-ordinates the training and education of the relevant specialty within an individual trust.

**Types of Assessments**

There are various systematic processes for measuring a learner's progress or level of achievement against defined criteria (including curriculum outcomes). This may be for summative or formative purposes.

Formative assessment: This assessment helps both trainer and trainee to identify the development requirements of the trainee and allows intervention to be made during the learning process. At present all workplace-based assessments (WpBAs) are individually formative. WpBA is a process to amass evidence of a trainee's progress in areas of professional practice. This evidence is recorded in a structured and systematic manner on a web-based portfolio (e-portfolio, see below). It is used to inform reviews and, at the end of training, to make qualitative judgement about the readiness of the doctor or dentist for independent practice. It provides feedback to the trainee and drives learning. There are many WpBAs, with some being specialty-specific and others generic across the specialties:

- Audit assessment tool—to assess a trainee's competence in completing a clinical audit through a written report or presentation.
- Teaching observation tool—to support and develop qualities as a medical teacher.
- Multi-source feedback (MSF)—provides judgement about behaviour and generic skills such as communication, team working and reliability within the clinical context. This assessment is completed by the trainee's peers, tutors and other members of the healthcare team to provide different perspectives about situations on separate occasions. The trainee will not see the individual response of the raters; feedback of the anonymised summary is given to the trainee by the Educational Supervisor.
- Direct observation of procedural skills (DOPS)—an assessment of performance in undertaking a planned procedure. The trainee receives immediate feedback to identify strengths and areas for development.
- Procedure-based assessment (PBA)—used in surgical and interventional radiology training (a detailed assessment for surgical/interventional procedures).
- Mini-Cex—a clinical evaluation exercise tool for assessment of a clinical encounter with a patient to assess competence in history taking, examination or clinical reasoning.
- Mini-IPX—in clinical radiology this is used to assess skills in interpreting imaging.
- Case-based discussion (CBD)—assesses the trainee's performance in clinical reasoning, decision making and application of medical knowledge in relation to patient care.
- MDT assessment tool—assesses the trainee's performance in a multidisciplinary environment which is relevant for future placements in acute trusts in secondary and tertiary centres.

The e-portfolio provides a developmental learning tool for trainees to plan, record and reflect on their training. It allows collection of evidence-based activities that the trainee has undertaken and is used to inform appraisal discussions and the ARCP.

Summative assessment: standardised examinations with a pass or fail outcome. All the Royal Colleges operate these exams, for example, MOrth (Membership of Orthodontics), FRCR (Fellowship of the Royal College Radiologists) and the MRCGP (Membership of the Royal College of General Practitioners), and they must be passed before practice can be undertaken unsupervised.

This summative assessment is how doctors conclude their specialty training and become members or fellows of their chosen Royal College.

### 8.3.2 Post-CCT Appraisal

Appraisal for specialty doctors and consultants is a developmental process using the framework based on Good Medical Practice. This framework provides a standard approach for all appraisals in which licenced doctors must take part in order to revalidate. The framework includes four domains (similar to those set out in the e-portfolio for pre-CCT trainees) which provide the structure to reflect on clinical practice and approach to medicine:

1. Knowledge, skills and performance.
2. Safety and quality.
3. Communication, partnership and teamwork.
4. Maintaining trust.

Peer review: This contributes towards the appraisal system for both trainees and specialist staff. It usually takes the form of multi-source feedback (covered in Sect. 7.3.1) from peers and other staff with whom the specialists work. In addition, the GMC requires doctors to submit patient feedback data for appraisal.

Post-CCT staff in the NHS also undergo a job planning exercise where the doctor's clinical and non-clinical activities are reviewed on an annual basis.

### 8.3.3 National Clinical Assessment Service

NCAS is a branch of the National Patient Safety Agency. It provides guidance and support to doctors, dental surgeons and pharmacists who are under-performing. It collaborates closely with the GMC, GDC, Royal Colleges and Trusts to provide a range of services from telephone consultations to full support, including one-to-one interviews and remedial solutions. Approaching NCAS is usually proposed by a senior member of staff such as the Medical Director, Chief Executive or one of the latter's delegates.

NCAS assesses and can manage problems relating to:

- health
- performance
- behaviour

Outcomes vary from simple remedial action to increased support, additional intense training and suggested exclusion from the GMC/GDC's registration list.

NCAS has been superseded by PPA, Practitioner Performance Advice. For more details, refer to Sect. 9.2.2 below.

## Further Readings

GMC (2013) Good medical practice. www.gmc-uk.org/Good_medical_practice___English_1215.pdf_51527435.pdf. Accessed Jan 2019

Health Education England (2016) Dental foundation training. Information handbook 2016–2017. https://madeinheene.hee.nhs.uk/Portals/13/DFT%202016%20handbook%20final.pdf. Accessed Jan 2020

Health Education England (2017) Supported return to training. https://www.hee.nhs.uk/sites/default/files/documents/Supported%20Return%20to%20Training.pdf. Accessed Dec 2019

NHS Revalidation Support Team (2013) Medical appraisal guide – a guide to medical appraisal for revalidation in England. www.england.nhs.uk/revalidation/wp-content/uploads/sites/10/2014/02/rst-medical-app-guide-2013.pdf. Accessed Jan 2019

The Academy of Medical Royal Colleges (2017) Return to practice guidance. https://www.aomrc.org.uk/wp-content/uploads/2017/06/Return_to_Practice_guidance_2017_Revison_0617-2.pdf. Accessed Dec 2019

# Clinical Risk Management in the NHS

# 9

## 9.1 Introduction

Clinical risk management is a very important aspect of healthcare. Every NHS trust in the UK has policies and guidelines in place to mitigate the risk associated with providing healthcare. Implications of deficiencies might impact the patient directly, family and friends accompanying the patients and members of staff. Clinical risk protocols are usually set up at a local level and further supported by national agencies. The latter are normally alerted to clinical events with serious consequences. The aims of the reporting set-up is to decrease the likelihood of a similar event taking place repeatedly.

Serious incidents in specialist tertiary centres should be directly reported to the NHS Commissioning Body. Incidents affecting mental health trusts should be directed to the Clinical Commissioning Group (CCG).

## 9.2 National Agencies

A number of national agencies listed below in alphabetical order are involved in clinical risk management:

- Clinical Commissioning Group (CCG)—streams funding to community, mental health and ambulance trusts. Investigate incidents that occurred within these trusts.
- Coroner—independent judicial experts, appointed by legal entities to investigate causes of violent, suspicious, unnatural or sudden deaths of unknown cause.
- Health and Safety Executive (HSE)—responsible for the enforcement of the Health and Safety at Work Act (1974).
- Local Safeguarding Boards—these are set up locally to protect both vulnerable children and adults. These boards are accountable to the board of NHS England.



S. Abela, *Leadership and Management in Healthcare*,
https://doi.org/10.1007/978-3-031-21025-9_9

- Medicines and Healthcare products Regulatory Agency (MHRA)—investigates serious incidents involving medication or medical devices.
- Monitor—investigates long-term financial sustainability of trusts.
- National Clinical Assessment Service—It provides support to NHS doctors and assists them by providing them with support to improve their performance. This in turn leads to improved patient safety.
- National Reporting and Learning System—a database containing details of patient-related serious incidents within the NHS. This database allows sharing of information to reduce the likelihood of similar incidents being repeated. The NRLS is managed by NHS Improvement.
- NHS Commissioning Body—streams funding to primary care, specialised care and investigates serious incidents.
- NHS Litigation Authority—manages and then settles financial claims including negligence claims against the NHS in England. Also circulates learning outcomes and attempts to prevent similar incidents from recurring.
- NHS Protect—Part of NHS Business Authority (NHSBA) with the main aim of investigating and managing any acts of fraud, corruption, bribery and theft amongst others committed within the NHS. It has been superseded by NHS Counter Fraud Authority in April 2017, an arm's length body to the Department of Health and Social Care. The members forming this authority are intelligence-led and have expertise at tackling and managing fraudulent matters.
- NHS Trust Development Authority—provides governance and accountability for NHS hospitals.
- Police—investigate incidents where there is evidence, or suspicion, of a criminal offence having been committed.
- Public Health England (PHE)—investigates incidents that might have the potential to affect the health of the whole population.
- Serious Adverse Blood Reactions and Incidents (SABRE)—the MHRA's online system for reporting safety incidents related to blood and blood components.

### 9.2.1 The NHS Commissioning Board Special Health Authority

See: www.england.nhs.uk/2011/12/designate-executive-directors/

The NHS CBSHA has, since June 2012, taken over the key functions from the National Patient Safety Agency (NPSA), and its key role is to deliver high quality and safe care to the public. The NHS CBSHA harnesses the power of the National Reporting and Learning System (see above). Patient-related alerts are streamed to the Central Alerting System (CAS).

**Central Alerting System**

See: https://www.cas.mhra.gov.uk/Home.aspx

Patient safety falls under the auspices of NHS Improvement which is also responsible for patient safety alerts (see Sect. 1.2.6 for more details). All patient safety alerts are published via the Central Alerting System (CAS) which is a web-based

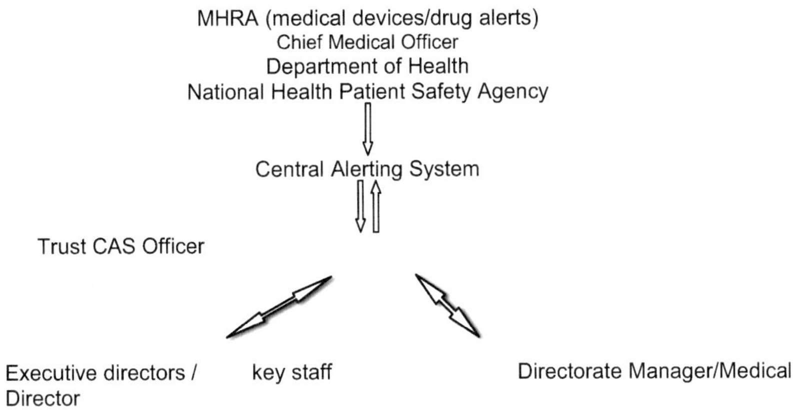


**Fig. 9.1** Flow of reporting between a trust and CAS

platform onto which concerns about patient safety can be raised and uploaded for viewing and increasing awareness. The CAS hosts safety information issued by the MHRA, the Chief Medical Officer, the DH and the NHPSA. Key personnel and front-line medical professionals can subscribe to email alerts and register to see the details of the alert online. Important public health messages, other safety-critical information, and guidance to the NHS and others (including independent providers of health and social care) are also uploaded on CAS (see Fig. 9.1).

The CAS issues three main types of alerts to ensure effective dissemination of new alerts:

1. **Rapid response reports**—for example the harm caused by flushing of nasogastric tubes before confirmation of placement (see full report at: www.nrls.npsa.nhs.uk/EasySiteWeb/getresource.axd?AssetID=133439&type=full&servicetype=Attachment—accessed January 2019).
2. **Patient safety alerts**—for example would be the risk of severe harm or death due to withdrawing insulin from pen devices (see full report at: https://improvement.nhs.uk/news-alerts/risk-severe-harm-and-death-withdrawing-insulin-pen-devices/—accessed January 2019). All patient safety alerts are continuously updated and uploaded on the NHS Improvement website: https://improvement.nhs.uk/news-alerts/?articletype=patient-safety-alert—accessed January 2019).
3. **Safer practice notices**—for example would be the early identification of failure to act on radiological imaging reports (see full report at: www.nrls.npsa.nhs.uk/EasySiteWeb/getresource.axd?AssetID=61469&—accessed January 2019).

In 2014, NHS England launched an improved alerting system with the aim of increasing the efficacy of disseminating new warnings and medical alerts to all treating clinicians. The new process allowed NHS England to publish monthly reports on trusts who fail to confirm they have complied with the required actions of an alert within the set timeframe. The new system consists of three stages:

- Stage One: Warning alert raises awareness amongst clinical staff as quickly as possible. This allows healthcare organisations to take immediate action.
- Stage Two: Alert provides detailed information and advice and offers access to relevant training programmes if needed.
- Stage Three: Alert requires conformity by all healthcare organisations to confirm adherence to approved checklists of required action.

### 9.2.2 The National Clinical Assessment Service

The NCAS was first established in 2001 and has been an operating division of the NHS Litigation Authority since 2013. It worked to resolve concerns about healthcare professionals (doctors, dentists and pharmacists), but it wasn't an investigatory body or a regulatory body. If concerns were raised about an individual, early communication with NCAS was vital to start any necessary support that the clinician might be in need of.

NCAS has now been superseded by Practitioner Performance Advice (PPA). Delivered by NHS Resolution, it aims at managing Healthcare Professional Alert Notices (HPANs). The latter are notices given in relation to safety concerns raised by suboptimal delivery by NHS bodies or healthcare providers.

PPA deliver the following:

- Clinical performance reviews
- Behavioural reviews
- Professional support and mediation
- Assisted mediation
- Team reviews

## 9.3 Serious Incidents

A serious incident is any adverse event with serious implications to patients, their families, staff and/or the public. A rapid response is justified to reduce the chance of recurrence.

### 9.3.1 Types of Serious Incidents

Serious incidents include:

- Acts or omissions in care that result in:
  - death
  - injury resulting in serious harm
  - injury requiring treatment by other health professionals to prevent death or serious harm
- Abuse
- Never events
- Incidents that prevent an organisation's ability to continue to deliver an acceptable quality of healthcare
- Incidents that cause widespread public concern, resulting in a loss of confidence in healthcare services

### 9.3.2 Management of a Serious Incident

Serious incidents must be verified by the trust immediately. The first steps are to:

- establish the facts
- ensure safety of patients and staff
- secure all relevant evidence to support further investigation
- take appropriate action

Serious Incidents (SIs) have to be reported on the Strategic Executive Information System (StEIS), which facilitates the monitoring of SIs between providers and commissioners. This in turn is reported to the National Reporting and Learning System (NRLS). NHS Trusts have this reporting system set up locally linking the reporting directly to the NRLS. If direct linkage is not possible, the authorised personnel would report it digitally via the NRLS e-form.

Serious incidents should be disclosed to the patient, their family (including victim's family where applicable) or carers as soon as possible. The healthcare service provider must be informed of a serious incident within 2 working days, as should other regulatory, statutory and advisory bodies, such as the CQC, Monitor or NHS Trust Development Authority. External agencies, such as the police or local authority, may also need to be involved depending on the incident.

The recognised system-based method for conducting investigations is commonly known as root cause analysis (RCA) and should be applied to all serious incident investigations.

**Root Cause Analysis**

This is a systematic retrospective method of analysing the root causes of an incident. The main questions that would need to be answered following the investigation are what, how, and why the incident happened. RCA is then used to identify areas for change and to make recommendations for sustainable solutions to help minimise recurrence of similar incidents. The key principle of RCA is to identify a wider cause for the problem rather than adopting a short-term approach simply to identify the cause for one specific incident. Systemic failures and issues, or root causes as the name implies, are assessed in an attempt to learn lessons and circulate information about these lessons to improve the quality of healthcare.

**Levels of Investigation**

The level of investigation should be proportionate to the individual incident:

- Level 1: Internal concise investigation—indications include less complex incidents which can be managed by individuals or a small group of individuals at a local level.
- Level 2: Internal comprehensive investigations—indications include complex issues ideally managed by experts and/or specialist investigators.
- Level 3: External independent investigations—indications include incidents where the provider or organisation cannot conduct the investigation without external input.

A Level 3 investigation should be considered for the following circumstances:

- A serious incident where the organisation is unable to conduct an effective and timely investigation.
- Deaths/near deaths of patients under the Mental Health Act (1983) with an unknown or preventable cause such as unsupervised self-inflicted death.
- The patient/patient's family have reason to believe that the care provided was deficient and that lessons can be learnt following an independent investigation to prevent similar occurrences.
- Multiple incidents represent a systemic failure leading to widespread public concern. A recent example of a systemic failure involved 14 paediatric surgery cases at Leeds Teaching Hospitals NHS Trust; an independent review for NHS England was commissioned. Concerns arose from three sources: mortality data, complaints expressed by families of children treated in the unit, and concerns relating to patient care expressed to NHS England from another NHS Trust.
- Failure of the services' configuration leading to serious incidents.
- Homicide by a person under care.

**Timeframe for Investigation**

Level 1 and Level 2 investigations should be completed within 60 days and Level 3 investigations should be completed within 6 months of being commissioned. The investigation is considered closed when the appointed commissioner finds that the action plan meets the required standard and can be implemented long term.

Figure 9.2 illustrates the general sequence of events following a serious incident.

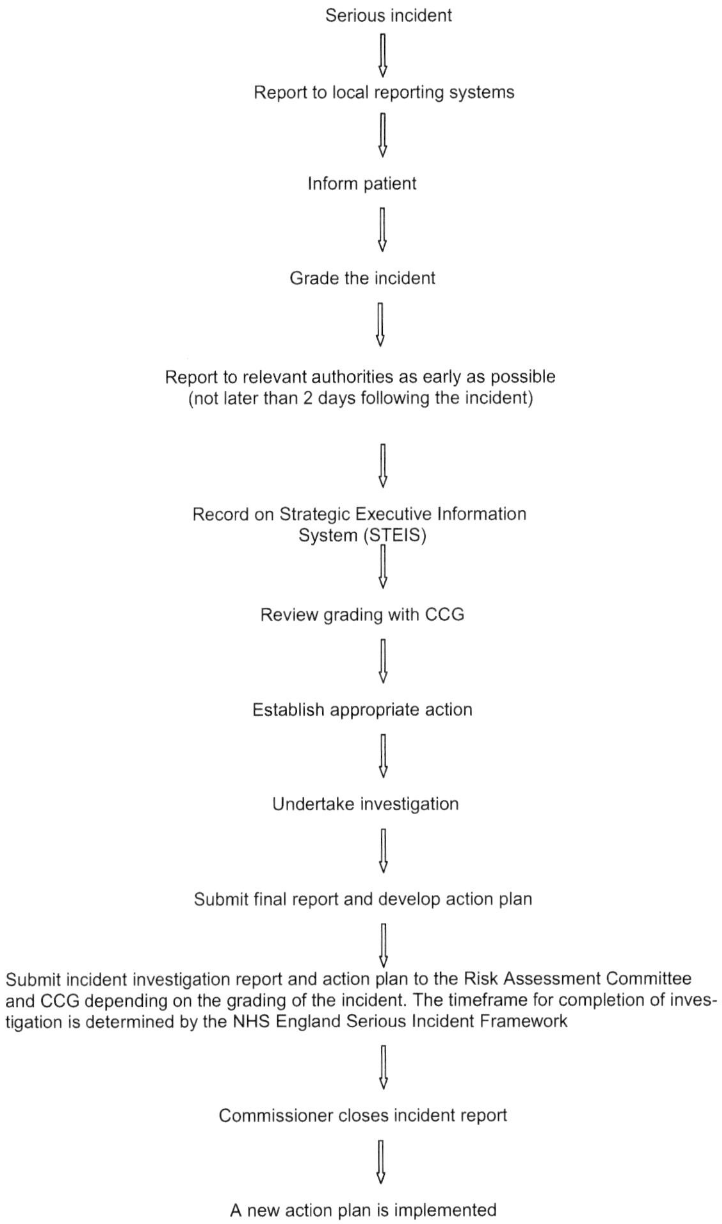


**Fig. 9.2** Cascade of events following a serious incident notification

## 9.4 Management of a Litigation Case in Acute Trusts

Each acute trust has a legal department that is usually involved in each litigation case. In addition, a trust will have a legal framework which needs to be adhered to when litigious action has been triggered (Fig. 9.3).

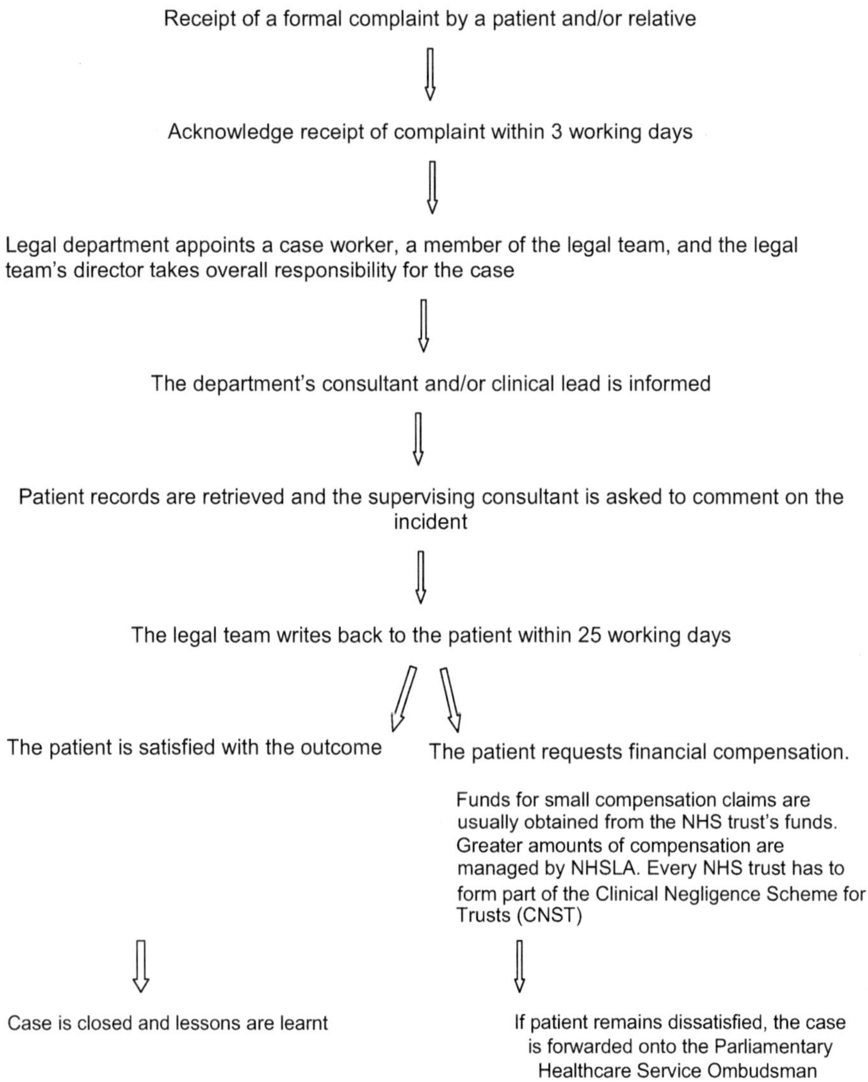


**Fig. 9.3** Management of claims cases in UK trusts

## 9.5 Risk Management Strategies in UK Trusts

Every trust has risk management strategies in place. Although they might vary between trusts, the principles are invariably very similar. Each trust uses a Risk Register and has a hierarchy to manage incidents depending on their severity (Fig. 9.4 shows a risk matrix for incident scoring).

Trusts employ 'being open' policies and every complaint, incident or adverse incident should be registered. Openness is regarded as safety and thus trusts registering more complaints are perceived as safer!

### 9.5.1 Risk Register Processes

The management of risk should form part of a doctor's training and so becomes ingrained into daily medical practice. Each trust has policies and protocols in place detailing the management of risks and/or incidences, and you should make sure you are familiar with these wherever you are work. Figure 9.5 shows a flow diagram simplifying the typical process in an acute trust.

| Severity | Likelihood | | | | |
|---|---|---|---|---|---|
| | Unlikely | Low | Moderate | High | Certain |
| No harm | 1 | 2 | 3 | 4 | 5 |
| Minor | 2 | 4 | 6 | 8 | 10 |
| Moderate | 3 | 6 | 9 | 12 | 15 |
| Major | 4 | 8 | 12 | 16 | 20 |
| Cata-strophic | 5 | 10 | 15 | 20 | 25 |

**Fig. 9.4** Risk matrix score sheet for incident scoring. Risk matrix score: 1–3 low risk; 4–6 moderate risk; 8–12 significant risk; 15–25 high/extreme risk.

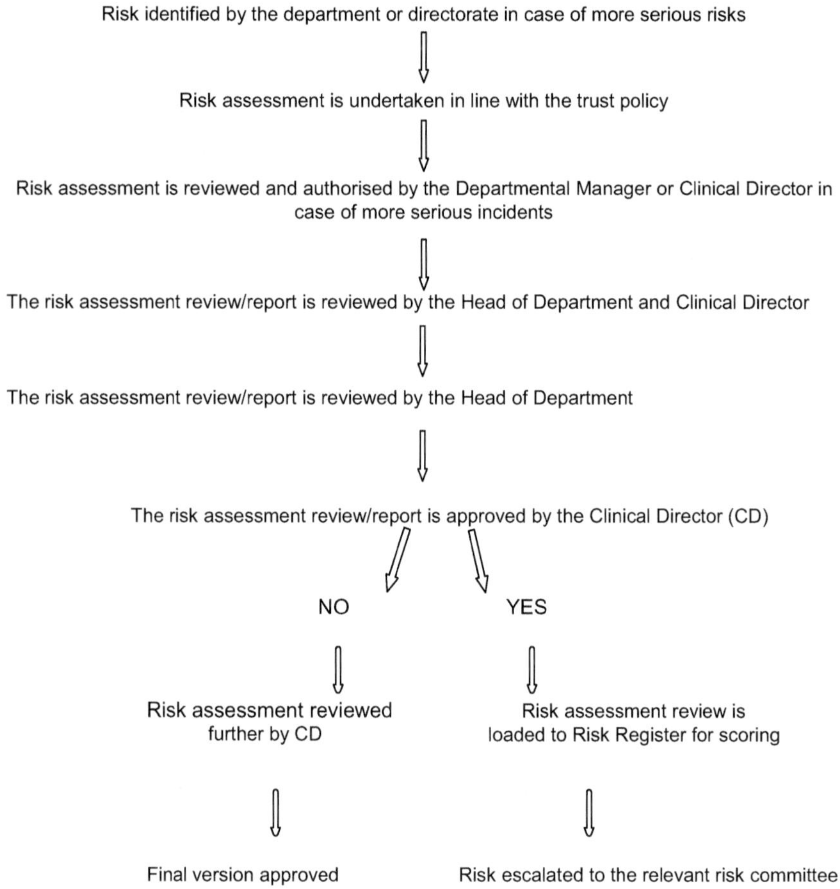


**Fig. 9.5** Pathway of risk management in NHS trusts

## Further Readings

Department of Health (2005) Independent investigation of adverse events in mental health services. https://webarchive.nationalarchives.gov.uk/20130124070128/http://www.dh.gov.uk/prod_consum_dh/groups/dh_digitalassets/@dh/@en/documents/digitalasset/dh_4113574.pdf. Accessed Dec 2019

Department of Health (2015) Revised never events policy framework. www.england.nhs.uk/wp-content/uploads/2015/04/never-evnts-pol-framwrk-apr.pdf. Accessed Dec 2019

Health and Social Care Information Centre (2015) Checklist for reporting, managing and investigating information governance cyber security serious incidents requiring investigation. https://www.igt.hscic.gov.uk/Resources/HSCIC%20SIRI%20Reporting%20and%20Checklist%20Guidance.pdf. Accessed Jan 2020

National Patient Safety Agency (2004) Seven steps to patient safety. https://webarchive.nationalarchives.gov.uk/20171030124342/http://www.nrls.npsa.nhs.uk/resources/collections/seven-steps-to-patient-safety/. Accessed Dec 2019

NHS England (2014a) An introduction to the NHS England National Patient Safety Alerting System. www.england.nhs.uk/wp-content/uploads/2014/01/npsas-guide.pdf. Accessed Dec 2019

NHS England (2014b) Independent review into concerns about paediatric cardiac surgery (the 14 cases) at Leeds Teaching Hospitals NHS Trust. http://webarchive.nationalarchives.gov.uk/20160605031147/https://www.england.nhs.uk/wp-content/uploads/2014/10/leeds-child-hrts-fin.pdf. Accessed Dec 2019

NHS England (2015a) Safeguarding policy. https://www.england.nhs.uk/wp-content/uploads/2019/09/safeguarding-policy.pdf. Accessed Dec 2019

NHS England (2015b) Serious incident framework. Supporting learning to prevent recurrence. www.england.nhs.uk/patientsafety/wp-content/uploads/sites/32/2015/04/serious-incidnt-framwrk-upd2.pdf. Accessed Dec 2019

Work Act (1974). www.legislation.gov.uk/ukpga/1974/37/pdfs/ukpga_19740037_en.pdf. Accessed Dec 2019

# Data Protection and Freedom of Information

# 10

## 10.1 Introduction

Legalities surrounding data capture are important and trusts can have fines imposed if these regulations are breached. Trusts place great emphasis on the need for confidentiality in respect of personal health data. This applies to manual and computer records, and conversations about a patient's treatment should be limited to between health professionals. Everyone working for the NHS is under a legal duty to keep patient information confidential.

Personal information, as well as health information provided by the patient, and added to by NHS staff, a relative or other person, must be stored securely.

## 10.2 Confidentiality Code of Practice

The Confidentiality Code of Practice of any healthcare institution, including hospitals, is usually found in the provider's policy and guidelines documents or the equivalent online platform. Health data can be captured in many forms including:

- digital format,
- transmitted via email,
- paper copy,
- verbal,
- recorded.

Sharing of information is only justified if this is of benefit to the patient and this should be restricted to the health professionals providing direct care to the patient.



S. Abela, *Leadership and Management in Healthcare*,
https://doi.org/10.1007/978-3-031-21025-9_10

Patients have a right to believe and expect that private and personal information which is given in confidence will be used for the purposes for which it was originally given, and not released to others without their informed consent. Sharing of information within the NHS requires adherence to Caldicott principles (see Sect. 10.3.3).

## 10.3 Data Protection Act 2018

This Act superseded the previous data protection Act from 1998. This Act makes provisions for more control over personal data held for added security and also makes provisions for the implementation of the General Data Protection Regulation (GDPR). NHS Institutions should ensure that they are in compliance with these regulations and enforces staff members to be knowledgeable of the rules surrounding the gathering, storing and sharing of patients' personal data.

### 10.3.1 Defining Personal Data

Personal data is information relating to a living person and includes any expression of opinion about the person. For a trust, all of the information held about patients and staff, whether electronically or on paper, falls within the definition of data prescribed by the Act.

### 10.3.2 Data Protection Aims

The Act in 2018 has adopted the following aims:

- Facilitate the secure transfer of information within the European Union.
- Prevent people or organisations from holding and using inaccurate information on individuals.
- Give the public confidence about how businesses can use their personal information.
- Provide data subjects with the legal right to check the information businesses hold about them. They can also request for this data to be erased.
- Give data subjects greater control over how data controllers handle their data.
- Ensures businesses are compliant with secure handling of personal data.
- Safe and secure storage of data. Data controllers must ensure that it is not misused.
- Require the data user or holder to register with the Information Commissioner.

### 10.3.3 Data Protection Principles

The Act in 2018 has adopted seven principles. These are as follows:

- Data must be processed lawfully, fairly and in a transparent manner.
- Purpose of data acquisition should be limited and for specific purposes.
- Data acquired should be minimised.
- Data held should be accurate.
- Data storage should not be kept longer than necessary.
- Integrity and confidentiality should be ensured during the storage timeframe.
- The data held should be accountable.

### 10.3.4 Caldicott Principles

The Caldicott principles, as laid down by the NHS Executive, must also be followed by the trust with regard to personal data.

- Principle 1—Justify the purpose(s)
  Every proposed use or transfer of patient-identifiable information within or from an organisation should be clearly defined, with continuing use of data regularly reviewed by an appropriate Caldicott guardian (usually a senior member of the trust's staff).
- Principle 2—Don't use patient-identifiable information unless it is absolutely necessary
  Patient-identifiable information items should only be used if there is no alternative.
- Principle 3—Use the minimum necessary patient-identifiable information
  Where use of patient-identifiable information is considered to be essential, each individual item of information should be justified with the aim of reducing identifiability.
- Principle 4—Access to patient-identifiable information should be on a strict need to know basis
  Only those individuals who need access to patient-identifiable information should have access to it, and they should only have access to the information items that they need to see.
- Principle 5—Everyone should be aware of their responsibilities
  Action should be taken to ensure that those handling patient-identifiable information (both clinical and non-clinical staff) are aware of their responsibilities and obligations to respect patient confidentiality.
- Principle 6—Understand and comply with the law
  Every use of patient-identifiable information must be lawful. Someone in each organisation should be responsible for ensuring that the organisation complies with legal requirements.

### 10.3.5 Differences Between the Data Protection Act 1998 and 2018

The main difference between the two acts is the limitation on international transfer of personal data. Safeguarding against deliberate international sharing should be in place via Binding Corporate Rules (BCRs) and Standard Contractual Clauses (SCCs).

### 10.3.6 Other Data Protection Principles

#### 10.3.6.1 Information

All members of staff should be informed about the trust's policies which should be available for access on the trust's intranet. There are rights to access personal data whether held in computerised or manual form and whenever the record was compiled. Ideally, encrypted storage should be used to ensure maintenance of patient confidentiality if the data is accidentally lost.

#### 10.3.6.2 Access

Access can only be granted following a written request accompanied by payment of a fee to the medical records department of a trust. Currently most trusts charge up to £40. A response to the request is usually provided by the data controller or the manager at the medical records department and the timeframe is usually approximately 40 days.

#### 10.3.6.3 Exemptions

For personal data about physical or mental health, there are two exemptions from the right to access:

1. where access to the data can cause serious harm to the mental or physical health or condition of the data subject or any other person
2. where the request for access has been made by another on behalf of the data subject and where disclosure is not permissible.

#### 10.3.6.4 Security

All data controllers (i.e. a professional responsible for holding patient-related information) must take appropriate security measures to safeguard personal data and ensure that a patient's right to confidentiality is not compromised. Special care is needed when sharing personal information to ensure that there is no infringement of the data protection principles outlined above.

#### 10.3.6.5 Research

Data processed for research or statistical purposes is exempt from certain provisions of the Act provided the processing does not cause substantial harm or distress to the data subject and is not used to support decisions about individuals. Such records are usually kept for 20 years although, if the ethical committee approves it, stored data can be kept indefinitely and becomes exempt from subject access rights if anonymised. The data subject should be informed of the intended use of the information.

There are eight general principles that guide Medical Research Council-funded research projects:

- All personal information is confidential and all researchers should obtain the patient's consent for their data to be used for research purposes, wherever practicable.
- All identifiable personal information should be anonymised in a form approved by the Research Ethics Committee.
- All personal information must be anonymised as far as is possible.
- Each researcher is responsible for any decisions to disclose any personal information.
- Researchers must ensure that personal information is handled only by authorised medical staff as agreed by the Research Ethics Committee.
- Principal investigators must undertake adequate training to prevent unauthorised breaches of confidentiality.
- Researchers must not be a cause of distress to patients.
- Researchers should make the research results readily available and publish them in the public database for a wider benefit.

#### 10.3.6.6 Maintaining Standards

Each year trusts complete an assessment of information governance standards and the results are submitted to the DH. These standards are usually included in the Information Governance Toolkit.

#### 10.3.6.7 Information Commissioner

An independent authority which has been set up to promote access to official information. A data protection fee to the Information Commissioner's Office (ICO) must be paid to adhere to the Data Protection regulations. This fee is applicable if you're a business, an organisation or a sole trader processing personal data, unless an exemption applies.

## Further Readings

Data Protection Act (1998) [www.legislation.gov.uk/ukpga/1998/29/pdfs/ukpga_19980029_en.pdf—accessed December 2019]

Data Protection Act (2018) [http://www.legislation.gov.uk/ukpga/2018/12/pdfs/ukpga_20180012_en.pdf—accessed January 2020]

Department of Health (2003) NHS Confidentiality Code of Practice [www.gov.uk/government/uploads/system/uploads/attachment_data/file/200146/Confidentiality_-_NHS_Code_of_Practice.pdf—accessed December 2019]

Medical Research Council (2000) Personal Information in Medical Research [https://mrc.ukri.org/documents/pdf/personal-information-in-medical-research/—accessed December 2019]

NHS England (2016) Confidentiality Policy [https://www.england.nhs.uk/wp-content/uploads/2019/10/confidentiality-policy-v5.1.pdf—accessed December 2019]

# Part II

# Management Scenarios

# Management of an Underperforming Allied Health Professional

# 11

**Scenario**

You are an ST6 trainee.

A nurse colleague approaches you and tells you that one of the junior doctors who recently started working in the department 'is no good at his job' and 'is putting lives at risk'.

What do you do?

## 11.1 Introduction

When presented with this scenario you will need to be able to discuss and expand on the following:

- underperformance,
- management of allied health professionals,
- knowledge of reporting to appropriate line manager,
- knowledge of trust policies.

The following flowchart provides an overview of the stages required.

Identification of a doctor's underperformance should always be followed by support and effective management in quick succession. Figure 11.1 below illustrates the management when managing cases involving underperforming doctors.



S. Abela, *Leadership and Management in Healthcare*,
https://doi.org/10.1007/978-3-031-21025-9_11

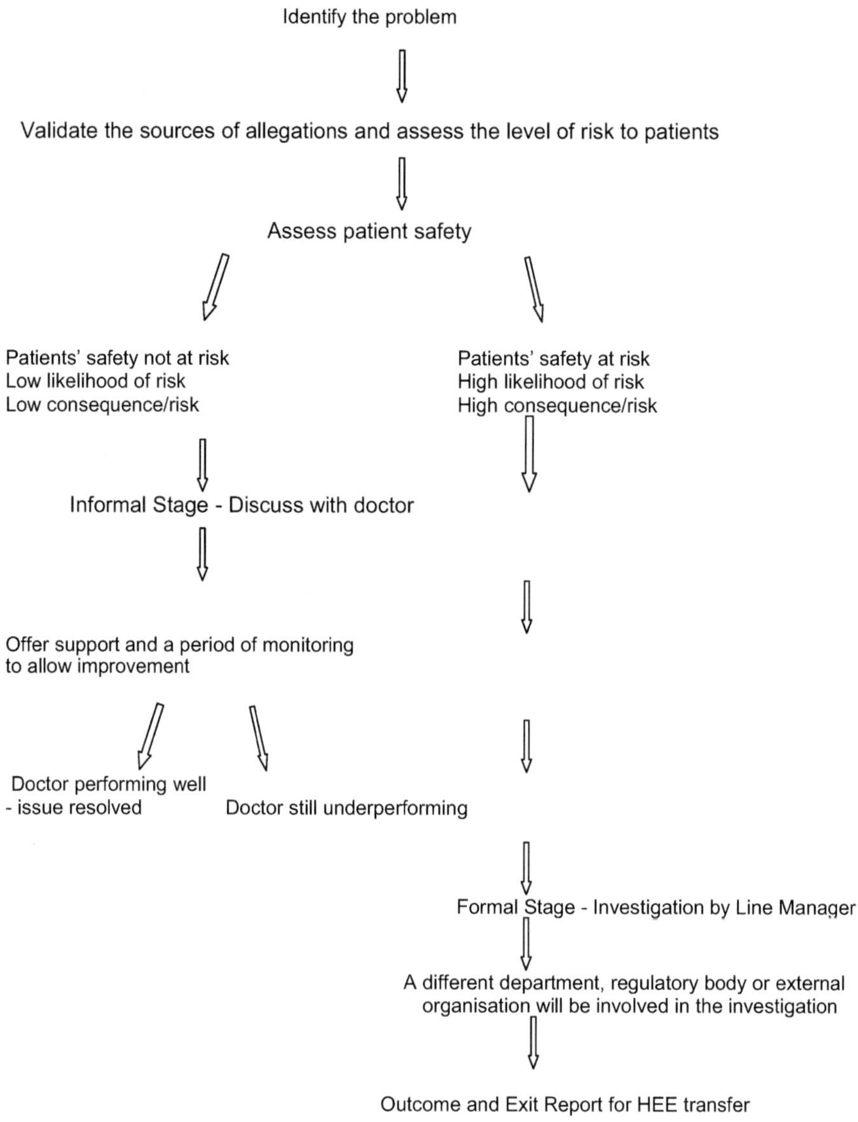


**Fig. 11.1** Flowchart illustrating staged management of an underperforming doctor

## 11.2 General Management Principles

The general principles in the management of poor performance, in chronological order are as follows:

1. Informal Stage—Identify the problem and work towards improved performance.
2. First Formal action—first stage of the formal process.

3. Final Formal action—second stage of the formal process.
4. Final Action—third stage of the formal process.

In stages 1, 2 and 3 the employee has the right to appeal and would be under observation to monitor the improvement in performance.

In most cases, guidance, training or advice will be enough to correct any ongoing problems. Depending on the severity and nature of the underperformance, a final formal action (a final warning) without first giving a formal warning can be warranted. This discretion may be used if, for example, the member of staff concerned is on probation, or if the underperformance is so severe that immediate action is needed.

1. The Informal Stage—Identify the Problem and Work towards Improved Performance

   At this stage, all the concerns are expressed and a personal development plan (PDP) can be set out. The consequences in case that no improvement is noticed are also discussed.

   Support, training and other appropriate help is offered and a timeline is set.

   The employee should continuously be informed of the progress and how the expectations are being met.

   If an employee's performance is unsatisfactory, discuss it with them after consulting with the appropriate Human Resources (HR) Advisor.

   Any causes for the underperformance should be scrutinised and the formal stage is only undertaken as a last resort.

   A note of the meeting is always agreed with the employee and a copy is given for their reference which is not included in their personal file but that the note will be included if a formal warning follows.

   In case of no improvement within the timescale set, the formal stages of the procedure have to be set up. Seven days of warning should be given with clear instructions that their performance has remained unsatisfactory.
2. First Formal Action—First Stage of the Formal Process

   At this stage, the employee is invited to a meeting and has the right to be accompanied.

   This will allow the employee opportunity to explain and/or offer solutions to the problem. The decision should be provided within 14 calendar days of meeting and it should contain the first formal written warning, with the employee having the right to appeal.

   A monitoring progress ensues stipulated in the outcome and if improvement is observed the warning will expire in 6 months' time. If no improvement is observed, the second stage of the formal process for a final warning stage follows.

   The employer at every stage of the process, depending on the nature of the underperformance and safety of the patients, has the discretion to give a final written warning without first giving a formal written warning.

3. Final Formal Action—Second Stage of the Formal Process

   At this stage, the employee should be invited to a performance meeting in writing, and has the right to be accompanied, with the employee given opportunity to explain and/or offer solutions. The employee is notified of the decision within 14 calendar days of the meeting where the final formal written warning is provided. The employee has the right of appeal and his or her progress will be monitored. This stage like the previous stage is a monitoring phase and feedback is given during the trial period.

   Upon improvement, the employee should be told about the 12 month duration of the warning.

   If no improvement is observed, a move is made to final stage of the formal process.

   An HR representative has to be present at this stage and the employee given a copy.

   The outcome of the meeting is put in writing and provided within 14 calendar days.

4. Final Action—The Third Stage of the Formal Process

   This is the final stage of the formal process whereby an employee is invited to a performance meeting informing them of a high probability of dismissal.

   In line with the previous stages, the employee has right to be accompanied and a full explanation is given of why the expected level of performance was not reached.

   With direct consultation with the HR Team, a recommendation is made to either:

   - extend the final formal trial period or,
   - transfer the employee to a lower pay band or,
   - dismissal.

## 11.3 Management Approach to this Scenario

The following approach should be undertaken, following the numbered steps below. An early and effective approach, coupled with the appropriate support, leads to successful management of underperforming doctors.

Step 1. Obtain information

When gathering information available it is important to consider the type of allegation and possible consequences, together with the quality of the information and then ask whether it is rumour-based or factual.

Important actions to consider:

- Classify the severity of the allegation into minor, moderate and severe and quantify the possible risk to patients.
- Inform other departments within the trust such as occupational health if the level of risk is very high.
- Inform his/her general practitioner for medical, physical or psychiatric support.

- Augmenting clinical monitoring to part- or full-time supervision of the doctor.
- Suspension from duties if risk to patients is high or there is grounds to substantiate the allegations.
- Informing the HEE providing their medical training.
- Informing the regulatory body.
- Reporting to external organisations such as the police, counter fraud authorities or security service manager in case of criminal allegations.

Reliable information can be obtained from:

- a professional colleague who reports the underperformance.
- examination of patient records completed by the junior doctor; this will allow an assessment of the accuracy of record-taking and precise completion of forms and investigations requested.
- number and nature of previous patient complaints against the junior doctor.
- performance review and/or appraisal records to assess the junior doctor's progress and/or any problems faced in the past.
- a clinical audit to establish the doctor's current practice compared to the gold standard; this audit can form part of the evidence that the doctor's performance is below par (the audit should be completed within a short timeframe so as not to delay the assessment).
- a regulatory body, or from a police officer or coroner.

The information should ideally be supported with written evidence and/or documentation.

Step 2. Assess Patient Safety

Ensure that there are no existing risk factors to patients, staff, members of the patient's family or to the institutional reputation.

Step 3. Informal stage—discuss concerns with the allied health professional.

Based on the nature of the allegations made, the feasibility of discussing the allegation with the individual needs to be assessed to verify or eliminate any inaccurate information. The examination should focus on determining the cause of the underperformance.

The best way to remember the various reasons for underperformance is to apply the following mnemonic and start answering the question by stating that this situation could be a reflection of multiple issues:

IF the PC is ProbLematic Switch to the Hot Desk:

Issues: Financial, Personal, Capability, Probity, Life events, Substance misuse, Health problems and Deficiency in training/education.

A report conducted by Harris R and Slater K, 'Analysis of cases resulting in doctors being erased or suspended from the medical register' 2015 has shown that all cases involving suspension or erasure from the general medical council register were due to personal or work-related incidents which are outlined below.

These type of incidents represent the most severe type of allegations made against a medical professional.

Types of personal-related cases were of the following types:

- sexual,
- dishonesty,
- drink-driving offences or,
- violent nature.

Types of work-related incidents involved:

- dishonesty,
- clinical issues,
- inappropriate relationships or,
- breaking other professional standards.

The total number of cases concluded in suspension or erasure, in 2020 were 147 and 92 respectively. For comparison purposes, erasures and suspensions, 5 years prior in 2015, totalled 119.

The line manager in turn informs the individual about the allegations made and then give them an explanation of your observations and any information you have obtained. The meeting should be prioritised without time delays and held privately to maintain confidentiality of personal matters. A period of monitoring of the doctor's work for 2–4 weeks (and occasionally for up to 3 months, if the allegations are very serious) should be agreed.

All line managers need to be informed about an allegation of underperformance by a member of staff, even if it is not serious and most probably won't undergo a more formal management route. All serious allegations that could affect patient safety should be formally managed according to trust policies.

It is essential that at this informal stage, the line manager:

- clarifies the nature of underperformance and the deficiency in comparison to the gold standard,
- fully explores the potential causative factors for the underperformance with the individual,
- agrees a new action plan outlining the remedial action needed with the individual,
- sets a timescale; typically not longer than 4 weeks,
- inform the underperforming doctor of the consequences should the deficiency not be addressed within the stipulated timeframe,
- explains the formal process if the performance target is not met,
- documents all of this accurately; underperformance, action plan, timeframe and consequences of not reaching the desired outcome.

Step 4. Review and assess following a very brief period (up to 4 weeks) of monitoring

The individual should be given a chance to improve, adapt to a new situation or allowances made to improve their performance to an optimal standard. The support that is offered to help the individual improve their performance and thereby conclude the informal process will depend on the nature of the allegation.

Following stage 4, the informal stage, the line manager should keep the individual up to date with his/her progress and no further action would need to be taken if the required standards are met. The records are retained for 12 months in the employee's file.

Step 5. Formal stage—Investigation if progress is not made.

A formal investigation is initiated by the line manager if the junior doctor in this scenario is unable to perform to the standards agreed at the informal stage. A meeting should be scheduled, with the individual given at least 5 working days of notice prior to the meeting. Any documentation gathered during the initial informal exercise could be utilised at this stage and will form part of the investigation.

### 11.3.1 Stage 1 of the Formal Process

Escalation to the formal Stage 1 will take place when the informal stage has not resulted in the required improvement in performance despite having being given initial, informal guidance and support. This stage may also be used in more serious circumstances the informal process might by bypassed altogether with a formal approach being instigated immediately.

A formal letter by the employer is sent to the doctor informing him/her of the formal stage of proceedings. This forms Stage 1 of the formal process and the following parameters listed below should also be outlined:

1. Confirmation of the formal stage of the underperformance policy.
2. Details of how the standards were not met.
3. Documentation of the doctor's underperformance.
4. Details of previous informal stage meeting including improvement standards care delivery agreed (if applicable).
5. Possible outcomes.
6. Timescale of investigation.
7. Relevant discipline and grievance trust policies.
8. Right to seek the relevant professional's body or trade union's or defence organisation's support.

The aim of stage 1 of the formal process is to provide further opportunity for the person under investigation to improve their performance. The formalisation process and letter forming part of this process should specifically clarify 5 of the factors listed above and are the following:

- Areas/duties of underperformance.
- Performance targets.
- Action plan.
- Time scale.
- Consequences of not obtaining the targets established.

The individual should present, in a meeting set up purposefully, any relevant reasons: work- or personal-related issues that were contributory to performance. The line manager would consider whether additional departments or external agencies need to be involved. The line manager at this stage of the process could discuss the options of redeployment or moving the timescale to allow sufficient time for the standards to be met. Timescales are usually set at 1 to 3 months. The remedial action required can be initiated or resolved through the internal organisation's departments and/or external organisations.

#### 11.3.1.1 Outcome of Stage 1 of Formal Process

The doctor should be informed that failure to meet the agreed standards would initiate stage 2 of the formal process with the possibility of not being able to continue his/her current post.

The doctor will be continuously kept up to date with his or her progress in line with the agreed strategy such as regular meetings and progress discussions.

Meeting the standards will allow the doctor to continue the contracted duties whilst monitored to maintain the standards agreed. Any records are kept for 12 months in the employee's file. If no improvement in the progress is noted, the line manager will initiate stage 2 of the formal process.

### 11.3.2 Stage 2 of the Formal Process

This is, as the name implies, the second stage of the formal process. It commences if the informal and stage 1 failed to improve the doctor's performance.

The line manager at this stage has the authority to schedule a progress meeting within 21 calendar days of failing to notice an improvement in standards as agreed from stage 1 of the process. A dismissal recommendation can also be released if agreed by the convening panel members which is set up by the line manager. In this case the panel will consist of the line manager, a senior manager with the authority to convene dismissal, a senior HR member and a representative from the regional HEE.

The doctor is given at least 5 days notice in writing. The letter should state the following:

- stage reached of the relevant discipline and grievance trust policy,
- details of how the agreed performance targets were not met,
- all necessary supporting documentation,
- details of any informal discussion and stage 1 outcome,
- right to seek the relevant professional's body or trade union's or defence organisation's support.

At this meeting, the junior doctor will discuss the reasons for the deficiency in performance with the convening panel and allow the doctor to provide any evidence that is related to the matter.

#### 11.3.2.1 Outcome of Stage 2 of the Formal Process

The chair of the panel determines the outcome of stage 2 meeting:

- can be satisfied with the performance of the candidate and reinstate continuous monitoring over 12 months to ensure that the standards are kept.
- can remain unsatisfied with the progress and issue a further monitoring period and a second formal warning.
- If the allegations are confirmed and are of a serious nature, the third and final stage might be skipped and the individual might be downgraded or dismissed.

The outcome of stage two meeting could include:

- A final warning.
- Retraining.
- Transfer to another unit outside the regional HEE.
- Downgrading to a lower banding.
- Dismissal on grounds of capability.

In case of disagreement, the interviewed doctor can appeal, following the trust's Appeal Policy.

### 11.3.3 Stage 3 of the Formal Process

This is the final stage of the formal process and takes place when the above steps have been followed and completed to no avail. In this case, the individual has not shown any signs of improvement. The individual at this stage would have been found not capable of continuing in the capacity in which he or she were employed.

#### 11.3.3.1 Outcome of Stage 3 of the Formal Process

At this end-stage of the process, dismissal is highly probable and the individual would be dismissed after consultation with the relevant HR and HEE teams.

In case of disagreement, the interviewed doctor can appeal, following the trust's Appeal Policy.

## 11.4 The Appeals Process

Every employee has the right to an appeals process.

The appeals procedure is as follows:

- The employee starts the appeals process by writing against the notice of dismissal, movement to a lower pay band or transfer to another post. This must be made in writing and within 7 days of the receipt of written notification of the decision. This appeal is heard within 14 days unless both parties agree otherwise.

The employee is invited to the appeal hearing and giving seven calendar days' notice, with the hearing normally occurring within 14 days of this notice.

Trade Union representation is allowed and opportunity would be given for presentation of any new evidence arising before or during the appeal hearing.

The outcome of the appeal hearing may include:

- confirmation of the original decision,
- overturning of the original decision and substitute a final or formal written warning,
- no sanction at all.

## 11.5 Trust Policies

Relevant trust policies that would offer a systematic approach to this situation are listed below in alphabetical order (the nomenclature of these policies varies between different trusts):

- Capability Policy.
- Disciplinary Policy.
- Equal Opportunities Policy.
- Grievance Policy.
- Medical Redeployment Policy.
- Patient Safety Policy.
- Sickness Absence Policy.
- Whistleblowing Policy.

# Management of an Injury Sustained at Work

# 12

> **Scenario**
> You are the clinical lead for a department.
> The ward sister approaches you to report that one of the healthcare assistants has tripped on a wire and injured her back. The ward sister also informs you that the healthcare assistant is in pain and can't work for the rest of the day.
> How would you manage this scenario in the short- and long term?

## 12.1 Introduction

When presented with this scenario you will need to be able to discuss and expand on the following:

- Risk assessment.
- Risk management.
- Knowledge of trust policies covering the management of risks and hazards.

### 12.1.1 Risk Assessment

This is a thorough examination of what in your work could cause harm to people so that you can assess whether you have taken sufficient precautions to prevent them.



S. Abela, *Leadership and Management in Healthcare*,
https://doi.org/10.1007/978-3-031-21025-9_12

### 12.1.2 Risk Management

Implementing and complying with robust systems in order to understand, prevent, monitor and decrease risks to patients, patients' relatives and members of staff. Mistakes should be studied to gain a learning experience and improve care.

### 12.1.3 Hazard

This is any individual thing that may cause harm to an individual or a group of people.

### 12.1.4 Risk

This is the chance of harm occurring to an individual or a group of people.

## 12.2 Management Approach to this Scenario

A trust policy outlining the management of an injury at work should be available as part of the trust policies section of your trust intranet. Senior members of staff or health and safety officers should be approached in case of doubt.

Figure 12.1 illustrates the management of an injury sustained at work in the form of a flow diagram.

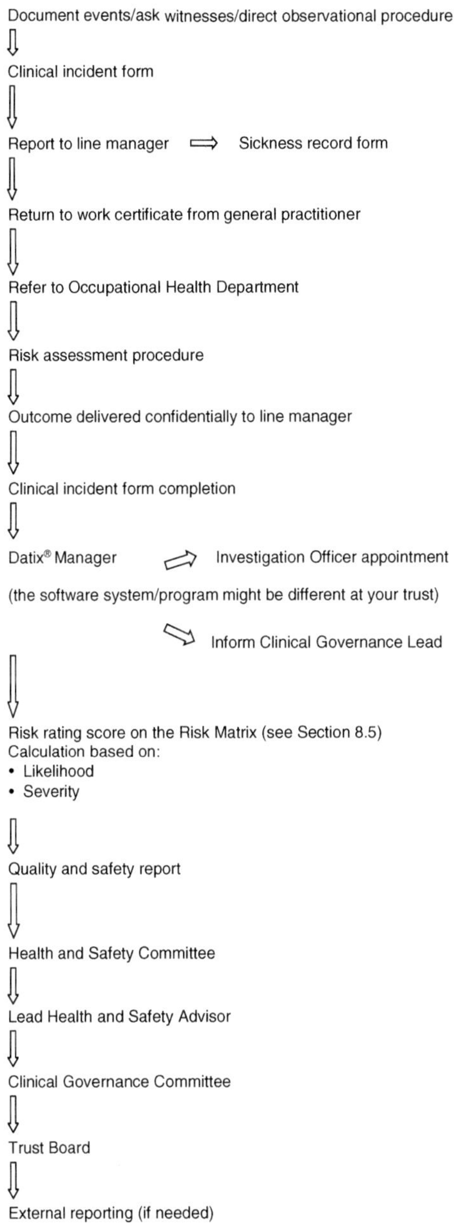


**Fig. 12.1** Flow diagram outlining the management of an injury sustained at work

## 12.3 Legislations

The relevant legislations that would apply to the management of this scenario are listed below (note that the nomenclature of these policies does vary between different trusts).

**Legislation:**

- COSHH—Control of Substances Hazardous to Health Regulations 2002.
- Health and Safety at Work Act 1974.
- Management of Health and Safety at Work Regulations 1999.
- Personal Protective Equipment Regulations.
- RIDDOR—Reporting of Injuries, Diseases and Dangerous Occurrences Regulations 2013, a revised version which superseded the version issued in 1999.

## 12.4 Trust Policies

The relevant trust policies that would apply to this situation are listed below in alphabetical order (the nomenclature of these policies varies between different trusts—make sure you are familiar with your local trust policies):

- Aggregating data and learning from incident's complaints & claims policy.
- Being Open Policy.
- Claims Policy.
- Complaints Policy.
- Consent Policy.
- Health and Safety Policy.
- Occupational Health Policies.
- Policy for the identification, assessment, recording and management of risks on the risk register.
- Policy for investigating incidents, complaints, claims to enable improvement and learning.
- Policy for the reporting, management and investigation of Incidents, near misses and SIs.
- Risk at work policy.
- Slips, trips and falls policy.
- Whistleblowing policy.

# Management of Clinical Incident at Work

# 13

**Scenario**

You are a consultant in the A&E department.

One of the nurses who works full-time in A&E has filled out a clinical incident form with regard to one of your junior doctors.

How would you manage this situation?

## 13.1 Introduction

The Patient Safety Incident Response Framework (PSIRF) is the NHS's strategy to maintain an effective system to decrease patient safety incidents and encourages an attitude to learn and improve on previously reported incidents.

PSIRF was launched in August 2022 and has superseded the previous framework—Serious Incident Framework (SIF). The former's publication intention was not to overhaul the existing system but to consider a patient incident and a serious incident as one that needs an equal response. The PSIRF is applicable to all members of staff operating within the NHS and includes ambulance, mental health and community health providers.

Each organisation should adhere to the framework and provide a policy and an action plan.

The former details the overall approach to patient safety incidents including the safety governance processes in place, the engagement of the affected individuals, the learning outcomes and the dissemination of these improvements to the wider organisation. The latter describes the methods and actions as the name implies the organisation takes to minimise the events from occurring in the future.



S. Abela, *Leadership and Management in Healthcare*,
https://doi.org/10.1007/978-3-031-21025-9_13

When presented with this scenario, you will need to be able to discuss and expand on the following:

- Clinical incident reporting.
- Management of clinical incident reports within the department and at trust level.
- Knowledge of trust policies covering these issues.

## 13.2 Clinical Incidents

A clinical incident is an event or an act of omission that has or may have resulted in actual or possible harm to a patient or group of patients. Clinical incidents should be reported to prevent repetition of the same incidents. The severity of an incident is based on the potential harm it could have or indeed caused.

Types of clinical incidents (in order of severity)

1. Near miss
   Any event or occurrence which, but for skilful management or a fortunate turn of events, would have led to harm, loss or damage.
2. Incident (sometimes referred to as an adverse incident)
   Any event or circumstance that led to unintended or unexpected harm, loss or damage. This can include physical or mental injury to patients, a member of staff, or a visitor, and covers both clinical and non-clinical incidents.
3. Serious incident [(SI) sometimes referred to as a Serious Untoward Incident (SUI) or Serious Incidents that Require Investigation (SIRI)]
   Serious incidents are events deemed to be sufficiently serious to warrant a formal investigation reportable to relevant Directorate/Partnership Senior Management with investigation monitored by the appropriate Health and Safety or Clinical Governance Forum. Usually they involve the risk of death or serious injury/ill-health, abuse, major damage to property, loss of service, or creation of a major health risk.

   Reporting serious incidents allows the appropriate identification and investigation work to be carried out. Lessons can be learnt through this process and these lessons can be shared to prevent the likelihood of similar incidents happening again.
4. Never event
   NHS England defines never events as 'incidents where there are or should be systems in place, at a national level, to make such errors wholly preventable'.

   Never events are serious, largely preventable patient safety incidents that should not occur if the appropriate preventative measures have been implemented. Whilst never events have the potential to cause serious patient harm or death, this outcome is not required for the incident to be categorised as a never event.

A list of never events is produced annually. The latest never event list for the period between the first of April 2020 to the 31st of December 2020 can be found at: https://www.england.nhs.uk/wp-content/uploads/2021/02/Provisional-publication-NE-1-April-31-December-2020.pdf—accessed March 2021.

The list includes:

- Wrong site surgery.
- Wrong implant/prosthesis.
- Retained foreign object post-procedure.
- Mis-selection of a strong potassium solution.
- Administration of medication by the wrong route.
- Overdose of insulin due to abbreviations or incorrect device.
- Overdose of methotrexate for non-cancer treatment.
- Mis-selection of high strength midazolam during conscious sedation.
- Failure to install functional collapsible shower or curtain rails.
- Falls from poorly restricted windows.
- Chest or neck entrapment in bed rails.
- Transfusion or transplantation of ABO-incompatible blood components or organs.
- Misplaced naso- or oro-gastric tubes.
- Scalding of patients.
- Unintentional connection of a patient requiring oxygen to an air flowmeter.

## 13.3 Management Approach to this Scenario

A trust policy outlining the management of a clinical incident should be available in the trust policies section of your trust intranet. Senior members of staff or risk assessment officers should be approached in case of doubt.

Figure 13.1 shows a flow diagram outlining the sequential approach for this scenario and Fig. 13.2 outlines the management options based on the severity of the incident.

The level of risk is ascertained by the Review Panel who have the obligation to report on STEIS within 48 h. If the SI is of a non-clinical nature, the responsibility lies with the Health and Safety Manager whilst if it of a clinical nature, the Patient Safety Manager will be responsible.

**Fig. 13.1** Flowchart for the sequence of events following a clinical incident report

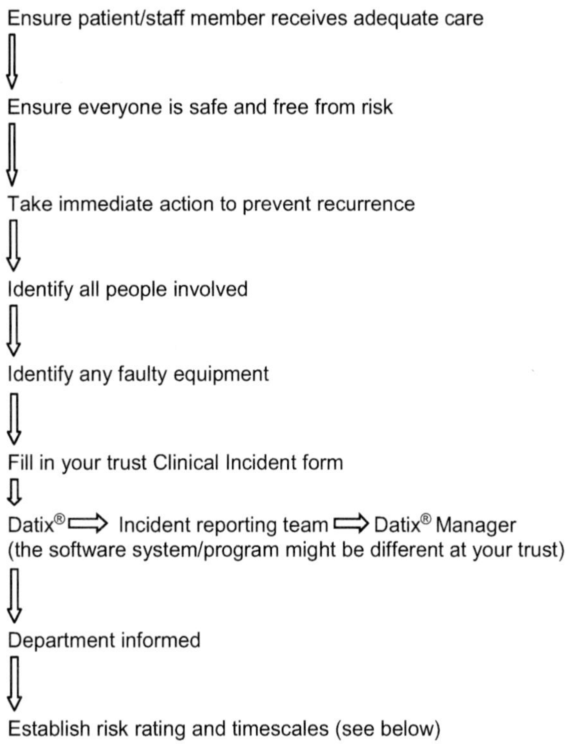


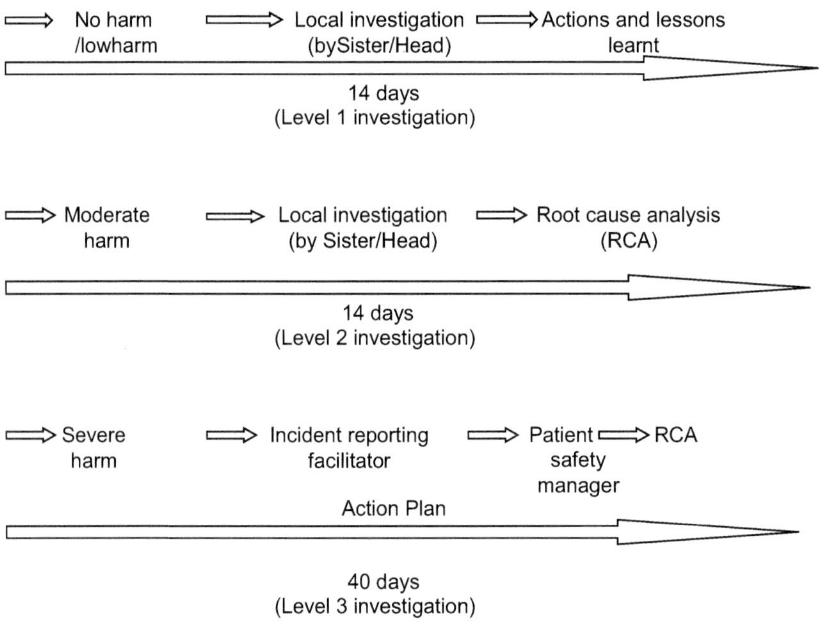


**Fig. 13.2** Management of clinical incidents depending on severity of the incident

**Table 13.1** External reporting agencies

| Types of clinical and non-clinical incidents | Responsible officer in the trust | External reporting |
|---|---|---|
| Radiation exposure | Lead IRMER officer | Care quality commission |
| RIDDOR | Health and safety team | Health and Safety Executive |
| Radiotherapy/any adverse incidents/near miss events | Incident reporting team | National Patient Safety Agency |
| Fraudulent claims | Incident reporting team | NHS litigation authority through legal services department |
| Medicine incident | Medical director | Medicines control agency |
| Medical device incident | Health and safety lead | Medicine health regulatory agency |
| Death | Head of department | Coroner |
| Violence/theft | Security manager | Police department |
| Information governance | Caldicott guardian | Information Commissioner's officer |

## 13.4 External Reporting

In case of serious incidents with serious ramifications, external reporting to the relevant agency has to be completed by a senior member of staff in the trust. Typical external agencies that could be involved are listed in Table 13.1.

## 13.5 Trust Policies

Relevant trust policies that would offer a systematic approach to this situation are listed below in alphabetical order (the nomenclature of these policies varies between different trusts—make sure you are familiar with your local trust policies):

- Aggregating data and learning from incident's complaints & claims policy.
- Claims Policy.
- Health and Safety at Work Policy.
- Human Resources Policies.
- Occupational Health Policies.
- Policy for the identification, assessment, management and recording of risks on the Risk Register.
- Policy for investigating incidents, complaints, claims to enable improvement and learning.
- Policy for the reporting, management and investigation of Incidents, near misses and serious incidents.
- Risk Assessment Policy.
- Risk Management Policy.
- Workplace Inspection Policy.

## 13.6 NHS England Legislations for Serious Incident Framework and Never Events

Below are the legislations published by NHS England with regard to serious incident frameworks and never events:

NHS England (2015) Serious Incident framework. Support learning to prevent recurrence [www.england.nhs.uk/patientsafety/wp-content/uploads/sites/32/2015/04/serious-incidnt-framwrk-upd2.pdf—accessed December 2019].

NHS England (2020) Never events 2020 [https://www.england.nhs.uk/wp-content/uploads/2021/02/Provisional-publication-NE-1-April-31-December-2020.pdf—accessed March 2020].

NHS England (2022) Patient Safety Incident Response Framework and Supporting Guidance [https://www.england.nhs.uk/wp-content/uploads/2022/08/B1465-1.-PSIRF-v1-FINAL.pdf—accessed September 2022].

# Management of Justifying Existing Levels of Care

# 14

**Scenario**

You form part of an Oral Health Consultant group in a department in one of the main teaching hospitals.

One of the members of your Integrated Care Groups (ICGs) approaches you to advise that NHS England will be reducing the funding that supports your specialty and shifting the funds to another area.

This would impact the provision of jaw correction surgeries that your firm can provide to the population within your hospital's catchment area.

How should you respond?

## 14.1 Introduction

When presented with this scenario you will need to be able to discuss and expand on the following:

- Knowledge of the new NHS structure.
- Funding streams and how your services can be affected.
- External support and knowledge in escalating the matter appropriately.

## 14.2 Clinical Commissioning Groups and Funding Streams

For further information about funding streams and CCGs, see Sections 1.1.1 and 1.2.5, respectively.


S. Abela, *Leadership and Management in Healthcare*,
https://doi.org/10.1007/978-3-031-21025-9_14

### 14.2.1 Funding Formulas

Funding formulas, mainly used by the now defunct PCTs (replaced by the CCGs), were a tool for distributing the centrally allocated funding equally and fairly depending on the geographical need. The weighting of these formulas was based on the size, age and level of deprivation of a population in a given geographical area.

### 14.2.2 Person-Based Resource Allocator

PBRA is a better method than funding formulas to produce more accurate estimates of a population health needs. This has subsequently been altered to give more weighting to age; this is referred to as ACRA after the committee that suggested its development (the Advisory Committee for Resource Allocation).

### 14.2.3 Current Allocation Strategy for CCGs

For 2015/2016 to 2020/2021 the allocation formula has the following main components:

- The general and acute need estimates.
- The mental health need estimates.
- The maternity need estimates.
- The prescribing need estimates.
- The Emergency Ambulance Cost Adjustment (EACA).

These allocations are subject to regular reviews to reduce inequalities in healthcare provision and target geographical deficiencies which could arise as a result of social mobility, a change in demographics and change in health trends.

## 14.3 Management Sequence for this Scenario

Step 1. Explain the specialism.

The first step is to explain the type of medical specialism that you offer, its mode of delivery and how the general health benefit from the specialty. Some medical specialties carry complicated nomenclatures and are closely intertwined with other specialties. Commissioners might not necessarily understand the type of delivery of care of your specialty to the population.

Step 2. Obtain background information and available guidance.

Past documents published and filed by DH are readily available online or upon request which provide information on historical collection of data about existing levels of care provision.

Step 3. Measure the new population's need for the type of care you provide in your region.

The contemporary need of the population will be measured against the current provision and funding can be adjusted accordingly. This can be done by measuring:

- The normative need by utilising official or qualitatively assessed indices. The normative need is based on the actual clinical need.
- The perceived need—this assesses patient perception of what it is necessary to treat.
- The treatment need which combines what patients deem necessary to treat with quality of life measures.

Step 4. Quantify the need for treatment.

The need, in this scenario, jaw discrepancies, needs to be quantified to allocate the necessary resources. In the UK, approximately 30% of the population need treatment. This information will lead to the establishment of an accurate figure of patients who need to be treated. The CCG in turn will allocate necessary funds to provide area-specific healthcare delivery.

Step 5. Establish primary care and secondary care providers.

Assess the number of eligible general dental practitioners (GDPs) with a special interest, specialist clinicians and consultants who might provide this service and also the number of specialists providing this service. Describe the existing structure available to patients accessing this type of care and how the resources are divided between primary, secondary and tertiary centres.

Step 6. Establish the community needs within your geographic area and assess whether there are inequalities between higher and lower socioeconomic areas with regard to treatment need.

Establish the geographical need for providing this service. Care should be tailored to meet specific demands in a geographical area and higher incidences of a particular condition should be managed accordingly.

Step 7. Match the need to the capacity after obtaining information about the numbers of providers.

Calculate the manpower available and then establish the possibility of providing the service at full capacity in order to reduce any potentially developing waiting list and provide care with maximum efficiency.

Step 8. Establish cross-boundary provision with providers from adjacent areas.

If the calculations in Step 7 show a deficiency of manpower, consider the option of attracting doctors from neighbouring areas or cross-referring patients to meet the demand. Establish the waiting times and structure of the NHS streams in your area.

Step 9. Draw conclusions.

Return to the regional CCG with factual information covering short-, medium- and long-term strategies to meet your local population's demands.

Step 10. Make recommendations.

Establish whether a reduction, or even an increase, in funding is appropriate.

Figure 14.1 illustrates the stages necessary to manage this scenario.

Define and explain the range of diseases/conditions that your specialty manages

⇩

Obtain background information and historic provision of care

⇩

Reasons/Justifications for providing treatment

⇩

Measure the new needs of the population

⇩

Quantify the amount of care delivery needed to improve the population's health

⇩

Quantify the existing providers in primary and secondary care

⇩

Assess the possibility of other providers that can supplement your provision

⇩

Make recommendations of whether the reduction in funding is justifiable

**Fig. 14.1** Justification of continued funding for treatment with the local CCGs (or in an interview-based question)

## 14.4 Further Reading

Relevant guides that offer further information on the CCGs allocation can be found below:


- NHS England (2019) CCG allocations 2019/20 to 2023/24 (core services) - guidance. [https://www.england.nhs.uk/wp-content/uploads/2019/01/ccg-allocations-2019-20-to-2023-24-core-services.pdf—accessed March 2021].
- NHS England (2019) CCG allocations 2019/20 to 2023/24 (primary care medical) – guidance. [https://www.england.nhs.uk/wp-content/uploads/2019/01/ccg-allocations-2019-20-to-2023-24-primary-care-medical-revised.pdf—accessed March 2021].
- NHS England (2019) CCG allocations 2019/20 t0 2023/24 (specialised services) – guidance. [https://www.england.nhs.uk/wp-content/uploads/2019/01/ccg-allocations-2019-20-to-2023-24-specialised-services.pdf—accessed March 2021).

# Management of a Suspected Victim of Physical Abuse

# 15

**Scenario**

You are a consultant in an NHS District Hospital.

A newly qualified foundation year doctor working with you on a new diagnostic clinic observes multiple bruises on the forearm of a 9-year-old girl.

What do you do?

## 15.1 Introduction

The safety of a child and/or adult should be the highest priority for any medical professional. In cases of suspected abuse, regulations governing the sharing of confidential information should be deflected in favour of the child or adult's safeguarding. Ideally, consent is always obtained prior to sharing any personal information, however, this should also be weighed against possible consequences if the child or adult is not managed and/or referred appropriately. The safeguarding officers within the organisation should be contacted to protect against further harm. The General Medical Council (GMC) provides a guidance to medical doctors. Further details can be found below with an online link to the guidance.

In most situations, when concerns are raised about the well-being of a child, the following steps are key to managing the situation appropriately:

- Consultation with a senior clinician or line manager.
- Direct contact with Safeguarding Team within the organisation.
- Referral to social services when warranted.
- Datix® Form completion.
- Full documentation of actions taken.
- Gain consent to sharing personal information with the relevant authorities.



S. Abela, *Leadership and Management in Healthcare*,
https://doi.org/10.1007/978-3-031-21025-9_15

When presented with this scenario you will need to be able to discuss the detailed management of cases involving abuse by expanding on the steps outlined above. This could be done by including the following details:

- Identification of child abuse.
- A comprehensive understanding of notifying the appropriate authorities.
- Safeguarding of children.
- Knowledge of trust policies.

## 15.2 Types of Abuse

There are four main types of child abuse:

- Physical.
- Emotional.
- Sexual.
- Neglect.

Types of abuse that might not be immediately apparent can include domestic abuse, online abuse, child sexual exploitation, female genital mutilation, bullying and cyberbullying, child trafficking, grooming and harmful sexual behaviour.

You should also be aware of fabricated illness; a rare type of abuse where actual abuse might not always be the causative factor. The most well-known example of this is Munchausen's syndrome: when a person acts as if they have an illness due to an emotional need. Munchausen's syndrome by proxy is where the parent or carer of the child exaggerates or causes symptoms of illness.

## 15.3 Signs of Child Abuse

It is imperative that a clinician can identify signs of child abuse. NICE has published a guideline describing the clinical features of abuse and neglect entitled 'NICE's guideline on child maltreatment'. The URL link to this document is found online: https://www.nice.org.uk/guidance/ng76/resources/child-abuse-and-neglect-pdf-1837637587141—accessed September 2022.

NICE has also produced guidelines on the following:

- Children's attachment entitled 'Children's attachment: attachment in children and young people who are adopted from care, in care or at high risk of going into care'. The URL link to this document is found online: https://www.nice.org.uk/guidance/ng26/resources/childrens-attachment-attachment-in-children-and-young-people-who-are-adopted-from-care-in-care-or-at-high-risk-of-going-into-care-pdf-1837335256261—accessed September 2022.
- Harmful sexual behaviours entitled 'Harmful sexual behaviour among children and young people'. The URL link to this document is found online: https://www.nice.org.uk/guidance/ng55/resources/harmful-sexual-behaviour-among-children-and-young-people-pdf-1837514975173—accessed September 2022.
- Domestic violence and abuse entitled 'Domestic violence and abuse: multi-agency working'. The URL link to this document is found online: https://www.nice.org.uk/guidance/ph50/resources/domestic-violence-and-abuse-multiagency-working-pdf-1996411687621—accessed September 2022.

### 15.3.1 Physical Abuse

Physical abuse can be defined as actions that deliberately hurt, or are intended to hurt, a minor by causing injuries. Physical injuries can include the following:

- Bruises.
- Burns and scalds.
- Bite marks.
- Unusual fractures or broken bones unrelated to sports activities.
- Other injuries and health problems.

You should bear in mind that child victims of physical abuse are unlikely to report the abuse, for obvious reasons. You are most likely to become aware of physical abuse through a patient's history such as multiple visits to A&E, for example.

### 15.3.2 Emotional Abuse

Emotional abuse is the second most common cause for minors to need protection from abuse and can be defined as ongoing emotional maltreatment of a minor. It leads to psychological damage to a child's emotional health and development.

Emotional abuse can include the following:

- Humiliating and/or constantly and unnecessarily criticising a child alone or in public.
- Threatening, shouting at a child or calling them names alone or in public.
- Blaming them for every single negative outcome.
- Forcing a child to perform degrading acts.
- Pushing a child too hard and showing no support.

### 15.3.3 Sexual Abuse

Sexual abuse takes place when an adult forces a minor to participate in sexual activities.

Sexual abuse can be: (a) contact or (b) non-contact abuse.

Contact abuse: As the name implies, contact abuse is the physical imposition of sexual activity on a minor/child. Examples of such abuse include touching, penetration, rape, and masturbation.

Non-contact abuse: Although there is no physical touching, grooming, online recordings, visual material and pornography could be examples of such abuse.

### 15.3.4 Neglect

Neglect is the lack of attention and complete disregard of a child/minor. This type of abuse takes four main forms:

Physical neglect—lack of provision of clothing, food and shelter.

Emotional neglect—lack of emotional support.

Educational neglect—failure to provide education.

Medical neglect—failure to provide the medical support needed such as failure to attend appointments.

## 15.4 Management of Child Abuse in a Clinical Setting

Figure 15.1 shows the sequential management of a suspected victim of abuse attending a clinical appointment.

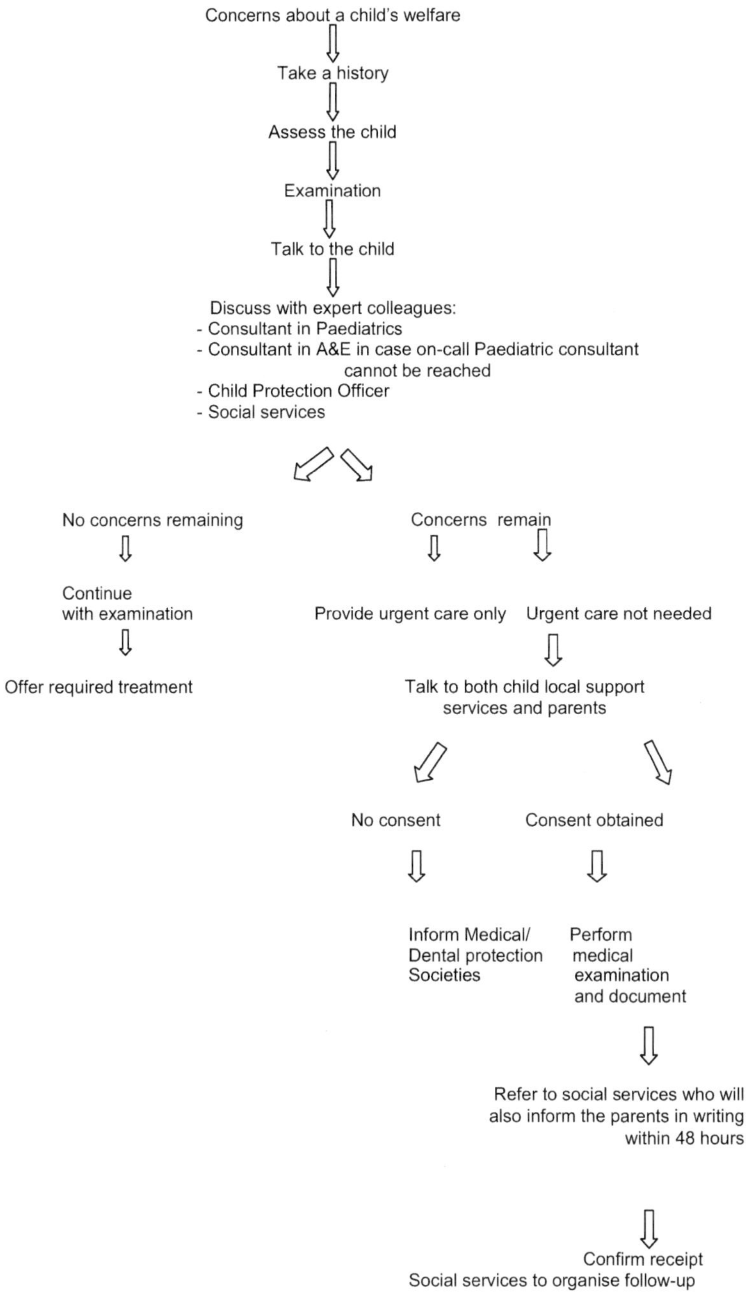


**Fig. 15.1** Typical management of child abuse

## 15.5 Relevant Trust Policies

Relevant trust policies that would offer a systematic approach to this situation are listed below in alphabetical order (the nomenclature of these policies varies between different trusts):

- Being open policy.
- Children who do not attend policy.
- Consent policy.
- Data protection policy.
- Digital images and recordings of patients' policy.
- Safeguarding children policy.
- Violence and abusive behaviour policy.
- Whistleblowing policy.

## 15.6 Legislations

Important legislations which are very relevant to safeguarding children are listed as follows:

- Equality Act 2010 [https://www.legislation.gov.uk/ukpga/2010/15/pdfs/ukpga_20100015_en.pdf—accessed September 2022].
- General Medical Council (2018) Protecting children and young people: A guidance. [https://www.gmc-uk.org/-/media/documents/protecting-children-and-young-people%2D%2D-english-20200114_pdf-48978248.pdf—accessed September 2022].
- Sexual Offences Act 2003 [https://www.legislation.gov.uk/ukpga/2003/42/pdfs/ukpga_20030042_en.pdf—accessed December 2019].
- The Children Act 2004 [http://www.legislation.gov.uk/ukpga/2004/31/pdfs/ukpga_20040031_en.pdf—accessed December 2019].
- The Children and Social Work Act 2017 [https://www.legislation.gov.uk/ukpga/2017/16/pdfs/ukpga_20170016_en.pdf—accessed September 2022].
- The NHS England Accountability and Assurance Framework 2019 [https://www.england.nhs.uk/wp-content/uploads/2015/07/B0818_Safeguarding-children-young-people-and-adults-at-risk-in-the-NHS-Safeguarding-accountability-and-assuran.pdf—accessed September 2022].
- Working Together to Safeguard Children 2018 [https://assets.publishing.service.gov.uk/government/uploads/system/uploads/attachment_data/file/942454/Working_together_to_safeguard_children_inter_agency_guidance.pdf—accessed September 2022].

# Management of a Breach of Data Confidentiality 16

**Scenario**

You are the head of a department.

You are told by one of the nurses at the start of a morning shift that one of your colleagues lost a hard drive containing confidential patient information.

What do you do?

## 16.1 Introduction

When presented with this scenario you will need to be able to discuss and expand on the following:

- What constitutes patient data.
- Consent to obtain patients' data.
- Secure storage of patient data.
- Knowledge of Data Protection.

## 16.2 Data Protection

By definition, data protection is the protection of personal information stored as data in paper or electronic forms.

The eight principles of data protection



S. Abela, *Leadership and Management in Healthcare*,
https://doi.org/10.1007/978-3-031-21025-9_16

Everyone responsible for using personal data has to follow strict rules called data protection principles. Individuals and companies must make sure the personal information is:

- Used fairly and lawfully.
- Used for limited, specifically stated purposes.
- Used in a way that is adequate, relevant and not excessive.
- Accurate.
- Kept for no longer than is absolutely necessary.
- Handled according to people's data protection rights.
- Kept safe and secure.
- Not transferred outside the European Economic Area without adequate protection.

The General Data Protection Regulation (GDPR) has been agreed upon by the European Parliament and Council in April 2016, and has replaced the Data Protection Directive in 2018 as the primary law regulating how companies protect EU citizens' personal data. As a result of the UK leaving the EU in January 2021, the UK has incorporated GDPR into its own data protection regulation. At the time of writing, UK GDPR and GDPR are equivalents, but you should keep up to date with any changes in UK law and practice.

The seven principles of GDPR are as follows:

1. Lawfulness, fairness and transparency.
2. Purpose limitation.
3. Data minimisation.
4. Accuracy.
5. Storage limitation.
6. Integrity and confidentiality (security).
7. Accountability.

Table 16.1 lists the principles of the Data Protection Act and the new GDPR showing the differences between the two.

**Table 16.1** The differences between the principles underlying the Data Protection Act 1998 and the new GDPR 2018

| Data Protection Act 1998 | GDPR 2018 |
|---|---|
| Fair and lawful | Lawfulness, fairness and transparency |
| Purposeful | Purpose limitation |
| Adequate | Data minimisation |
| Accurate | Accuracy |
| Retention | Storage limitation |
| Rights | (no equivalent principle) |
| Security | Integrity and confidentiality |
| International transfer | (no equivalent principle) |
| (No equivalent GDPR principle) | Accountability |

### 16.2.1 Obtaining Consent

The document '12 key points on consent: the law in England', published by the DH, contains the key points that a clinician should be aware of when practising in the UK. The GMC published a guidance document entitled: 'Consent: patients and doctors making decisions together' and the GDC published a document entitled 'The principles of patient consent', which similarly outlines the legal framework forming the basis of the consent process.

In daily practice, if in any doubt, the best practice would be to consult the Caldecott Guardian within the trust.

Photographs are a common form of graphical media that doctors ask for. They form a baseline record, especially if the condition is being monitored long term. Photographs enable comparison and illustrate changes in the condition/lesion between different time frames. Patients would be asked for consent of photographs and their use thereafter. Consent is taken by the doctor and reconfirmed by the person obtaining the records. The consent can be obtained on the request form or online if the latter is set up. For photographs, the doctor should obtain the following types of consent:

- Full consent for use of the graphical media (e.g. dermatological photographs) for teaching and medical publications.
- Consent for use of graphical media for teaching only.
- Consent to place the graphical media in the patient medical records.

### 16.2.2 When Is Consent Not Necessary?

Consent is not needed when a patient is not identifiable through the images. Such instances include images of histopathology slides, ultrasound views, radiographs and images of laparoscopic views.

Other bodies relevant to managing patient-identifiable data.

### 16.2.3 The Information Commissioner's Office (ICO)

Website: www.ico.org.uk

The ICO is a non-departmental public body that reports to parliament and is sponsored by the Department of Digital, Media, Culture and Sport. Each organisation handling PID should be registered with ICO.

The ICO was set up to uphold information rights in the public interest promoting openness by public bodies. The Data Protection Act 1998 states that every data controller, a member of staff within the organisation or health authority, that processes individual and personal information, should be a member of ICO.

### 16.2.4 The National Information Governance Board for Health and Social Care (NIGB)

Archived Website: http://webarchive.nationalarchives.gov.uk/20130513181011/http://www.nigb.nhs.uk/

The functions of NIGB have been transferred to CQC—Care Quality Commission.

CQC suggests the use of the NHS Digital Data Security and Protection Toolkit to assess the degree of adherence to GDPR. The toolkit should be adopted by all care providers that work under the NHS Standard Contract. Access to the Data Security and Protection Toolkit can be accessed online via: https://www.dsptoolkit.nhs.uk

### 16.2.5 UK Caldicott Guardian Council

Website: https://www.ukcgc.uk

The group's function is to provide support to the national Caldicott Guardians. They are encouraged to follow the Caldecott Guardian principles and a manual for all guardians has also been launched by the group to serve as a reference.

The web version of the Manual for Caldicott Guardians can be accessed by clicking the following URL:

https://assets.publishing.service.gov.uk/government/uploads/system/uploads/attachment_data/file/581213/cgmanual.pdf—accessed December 2019.

## 16.3 Management of Loss of Patient Identifiable Data

Management of loss of patient identifiable data (PID) is considered to be a serious incident and has to be escalated to the organisation's Information Governance Officer (IGO), Senior Information Governance Officer (SIGO) or Risk Officer (RO). The organisation's CG is responsible for ensuring and safeguarding the PID.

Referring back to the scenario, the first thing to establish is exactly what data has been lost, and confirm that the data is PID. If the data is patient identifiable data, then this is considered a serious incident. If the patient's identifiable data is not lost or the data cannot be associated or proven to belong to a specific patient, the risk is registered at a lower level.

Figure 16.1 shows a flow diagram illustrating the management of such a scenario.

Report of loss and/or theft of PID to your Line Manager

⇓

Inform Head of Department

⇓

File a Clinical Incident report online on the intranet

⇓

Report incident to the Clinical Director, police department (if theft is suspected) and the organisation's Caldicott Guardian

⇓

Measure Risk Score
Refer to the Appendix section for calculation of the risk score

⇓

Initiate investigation into loss

⇓

Alert and inform affected patients

⇓

Put measures in place to prevent incident recurring

⇓

Follow the new protocol issued by the trust (if changes have been made) for safeguarding PID to all members of staff

**Fig. 16.1** Flow diagram for the management of loss of PID

## 16.4 Legislation and Typical Trust Policies

The following legislations, policies and guidance are very relevant for the security of PID:

Data Protection Act 1998 [https://www.legislation.gov.uk/ukpga/1998/29/pdfs/ukpga_19980029_en.pdf—accessed December 2019].
Data Protection Act 2018 [http://www.legislation.gov.uk/ukpga/2018/12/pdfs/ukpga_20180012_en.pdf—accessed December 2019].

**Policies:**

Department of Health (2001) 12 key points on consent: the law in England [http://www.wales.nhs.uk/Publications/keypoints-e.pdf—accessed February 2018]

NHS England (2016) Confidentiality Policy [https://www.england.nhs.uk/wp-content/uploads/2019/10/confidentiality-policy-v5.1.pdf—accessed December 2019]

**Guidance:**

General Dental Council (2013). Standards for the Dental Team [https://standards.gdc-uk.org/Assets/pdf/Standards%20for%20the%20Dental%20Team.pdf—accessed January 2020].

General Medical Council (2013) Good Medical Practice [https://www.gmc-uk.org/-/media/documents/Good_medical_practice___English_1215.pdf_51527435.pdf—accessed December 2019].

# Management of a Formal Complaint 17

**Scenario**
You are a consultant.
The trust's legal department sends you a letter requesting the records of a patient you have been treating over the last 3 years. You find out that she has formally complained to the trust about the treatment you provided.
What do you do?

## 17.1 Introduction

When presented with this scenario you will need to be able to discuss and expand on the following:

- Types of complaints.
- How to manage complaints.
- Knowledge of the trust's structure regarding the management of complaints.

All medical professionals' first point of contact when a complaint arises, is their indemnity provider.

In England, all hospital-based medical doctors including locum doctors are covered through the Clinical Negligence Scheme for Trusts (CNST). In Wales, this is provided by the Welsh Risk Pool Services, whilst for Scotland this is provided by the Clinical Negligence and Other Risks Indemnity Scheme. In Northern Ireland each trust provides indemnity.



S. Abela, *Leadership and Management in Healthcare*,
https://doi.org/10.1007/978-3-031-21025-9_17

As from the 1st of April 2019, GPs providig care within the NHS in England, will have their indemnity covered provided through the Clinical Negligence Scheme for GPs (CNSGP) which is administered by NHS Resolution. In Wales, the General Medical Practice Indemnity (GMPI) scheme will provide this cover while in Scotland this type of provision for cover has still not been established.

Private-practice-based hospital doctors and general practitioners are legally required to possess personally arranged medical indemnity.

Medical Defence Organisations (MDOs) are mutual non-profit making organisations, owned by their paying members, the registered healthcare workers.

The primary function of MDOs is to indemnify doctors for incidents arising from their clinical care of patients and to provide members with 24-h access to advice and assistance on medico–legal issues arising from clinical practice.

There are three MDOs:

- Medical Defence Union (MDU)
- Medical Protection Society (MPS)
- Medical and Dental Defence Union of Scotland (MDDUS)

In addition to the above-three mentioned MDOs, a number of private companies also provide indemnity cover.

All medical professionals should ensure they have a minimum personal liability cover which is reviewed annually.

## 17.2 Complaints

**Who can complain?**

Any single individual or group of people who have been affected by an action or act of omission, neglect or decision taken on behalf of the trust.

A complaint may also be submitted by the patient's friend or a family member or anyone who has responsibility for the patient's welfare.

A number of external bodies or agencies may be used by patients to help them to put a complaint forward:

- Advice Now
- AVMA—Action Against Medical Accidents
- BDA—British Dental Association
- BMA—British Medical Association

- NHS Complaints Service
- NHS Direct
- Patients Association Forum
- Patient UK

**Main methods of complaining**

There are three main methods by which a complaint can be made:

1. By writing to the Chief Executive of the trust or the Legal and Complaints Department.
2. By liaising with the Patient Advisory and Liaison Services (PALS).
3. Online—trust websites have a dedicated section for complaints.

**Information to include in the complaint**

The letter should specify:

- The department where treatment has been carried out.
- The clinicians/healthcare staff involved.
- Timescales.
- Any grievances experienced.
- Ideal outcome to be achieved by triggering the complaint process.

Delegates authorised to handle complaints

All complaints are handled by the Trust's Legal Services Department

**Timescales for complaint handling**

The following timescales apply:

Time limit for the patient and/or family member and/or friend to make a complaint: 12 months from the incident date.

Time limit for the trust to acknowledge receipt of a complaint: 3 days.

Time limit for complaint to be investigated: 25 working days (1 month approximately).

The complainant can be expected to be kept up to date and should it be necessary to extend the normally agreed 25 working day target, an update should be provided every 10 working days. This can be done by any means of communication, but should be agreed with the complainant.

If a response is not provided within 6 months from the date of the complaint, the institution must write to the complainant explaining the reason for the delay.

**Contents of the Response**

The response should include the following details:

- An explanation of how the complaint has been considered.
- An apology if appropriate.
- An explanation based on facts.
- Whether the complaint in full or in part has been validated.
- The conclusions reached in relation to the complaint include any remedial action that the organisation considers to be appropriate.
- Confirmation that the organisation will take the necessary action/s.
- Dissemination of lessons learnt and ways how the trust will minimise the chances of similar events happening again.
- Information and contact details of the Parliamentary and Health Service Ombudsman in case the complainant is not satisfied with the response given by the local trust.

## 17.3 Management of a Complaint

Figure 17.1 provides a sequential process for the handling of complaints.

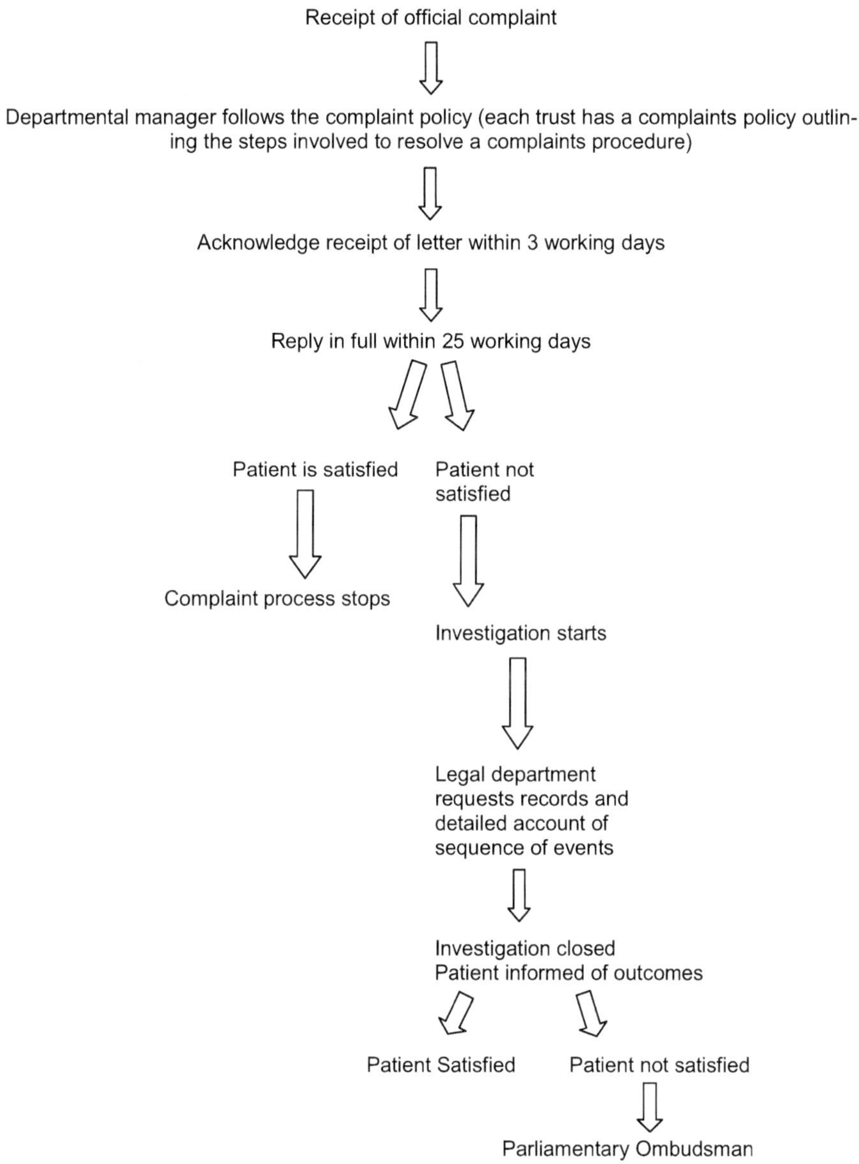


**Fig. 17.1** A typical complaint process

## 17.4 Taking the Complaint Further

If the patient is not satisfied with the outcome of the complaints process, they can appeal to the Parliamentary and Health Services Ombudsman and NHS Resolution.

**Parliamentary and Health Service Ombudsman**
The PHSO (www.ombudsman.org.uk) handles complaints that have already been assessed by the trust first. If the complainant is not happy with the first outcome, further opportunities should be given by the trust including the involvement of an independent conciliator. Once all the reconciliation paths have been explored and the complainant is still dissatisfied, the PHSO can be involved. The PHSO does not process any financial matters. They can be contacted by phone on 03450154033 or by email at phso.enquiries@ombudsman.org.uk. The Ombudsman will only seek to resolve matters once all local efforts have been exploited by the local trust.

**The NHS Litigation Authority**
The NHS LA (www.nhsla.com/Pages/Home.aspx) investigates and compensates patients pursuing a financial claim against the individual or trust.

**The NHS Resolution**
In April 2017, NHS LA was superseded by NHS Resolution, an arm's length body of the DH. The online webpage for NHS Resolution can be accessed via:

https://resolution.nhs.uk/about/

The NHS Resolution handles negligence claims made against the NHS institutions and independent healthcare providers of NHS care in England, through an annual membership. It obtains funding contributions from all NHS bodies and acts as an insurer.

Any claims are processed via an online portal.

NHS Resolution also handles concerns about the performance of doctors, a service taken over from the former National Clinical Assessment Service and disputes between primary care contractors and NHS England which was formerly managed by the Family Health Services Appeal Unit.

NHS Resolution will get involved if the Parliamentary Ombudsman makes recommendations against a claim due to injustice. Payments made by organisations may be eligible for full or partial reimbursement by NHS Resolution.

## 17.5 Legislation and Typical Trust Policies

Three important legislations that are very relevant to processing of complaints are the following:

- Freedom of Information Act 2000
- Health Care and Associated Professions (Indemnity Arrangements) Order 2014
- Public Interest Disclosure Act 1998

Relevant trust policies that would offer a systematic approach to this situation are listed below in alphabetical order (the nomenclature of these policies varies between different trusts):

- Being Open Policy
- Claims Management Policy
- Complaints Policy
- Incident Reporting Policy

## Further Reading

NHS England (2017) NHS England Complaints Policy, June 2017. https://www.england.nhs.uk/wp-content/uploads/2016/07/nhse-complaints-policy-june-2017.pdf. Accessed Aug 2019

NHS Resolution (2017) Reporting Claims to NHS Resolution, June 2017. https://resolution.nhs.uk/wp-content/uploads/2018/09/NHS-Resolution-Claims-reporting-guidelines.pdf. Accessed Dec 2019

# Management of a Contaminated Needlestick Injury

# 18

**Scenario**

You are one of the department's permanent members of the medical staff.

A staff nurse has a sharps injury after taking a blood sample from a patient who is a known drug user.

What do you do?

## 18.1 Introduction

When presented with this scenario you will need to be able to discuss and expand on the following:

- Knowledge of health and safety regulations.
- Knowledge of cross-infection policies and protocols.
- Adherence to mandatory training by all members of staff.
- Compliance with induction training, and continuous updating of skills and cross-infection procedures.

## 18.2 Incidence of Needlestick Injuries

Needlestick injuries are one of the most common injuries to affect NHS works, accounting for around 17% of all reported injuries.



S. Abela, *Leadership and Management in Healthcare*,
https://doi.org/10.1007/978-3-031-21025-9_18

## 18.3 Needlestick Injuries and Blood-Borne Pathogens

Any blood-borne pathogen is of concern of course, but the three major blood-borne viruses that are of particular concern to healthcare workers are:

- Hepatitis B virus (HBV)
- Hepatitis C virus (HCV)
- Human immunodeficiency virus (HIV)

**Considerations in case of HBV, HCV or HIV exposure**
History of vaccination
Need for a booster dose
Previous immunisation levels (HBsAB)
New blood screening test

**Risk Assessment**
Percutaneous exposure involving fresh blood from an infected source:

| | |
|---|---|
| Hepatitis B virus | 1 in 3 |
| Hepatitis C virus | 1 in 30 |
| Human immunodeficiency virus | 1 in 300 |

Percutaneous exposure involving fresh blood from an unknown source:

| | |
|---|---|
| Hepatitis B virus | 1 in 100 |
| Hepatitis C virus | 1 in 300 |
| Human immunodeficiency virus | 1 in 30,000 |

Every trust screens healthcare workers before starting a new post and records the presence of any potential transmissible pathogenic disease. This allows recording of the potential risk of possible pathogens being transmitted. An employee can start a new position once clearance from the occupational health department is achieved.

## 18.4 Reducing the Risk of Transition

**Reducing the risk of transmission**
The risk of transmission of viruses should be carefully monitored by both the employer and the healthcare worker.

Responsibility for Monitoring: Lead Health and Safety Advisor.

Monitoring Mechanism: Internal Health and Safety Department. Audits are routinely carried out to ensure safety is maintained such as adequate distribution and collection of sharps bins.

Responsible committee: The Health and Safety Committee provides all the reporting arrangements.

Table 18.1 lists the precautions and actions that need to be taken by both parties involved.

**Table 18.1** Trust and employee responsibilities to decrease blood-borne virus transmission

| Employer | Employee |
|---|---|
| Formal risk assessment | Compliance with immunisations and boosters as required |
| Provision of training | Personal protective equipment to be worn at all times, including gloves and eye protection<br>Maintain up-to-date medical knowledge and obtain adequate training |
| Provision of safe and protective equipment | Safe needles should be used; no re-sheathing should be permitted<br>Needles and any sharp objects should be discarded appropriately |
| Establish a local reporting system via Occupational Health department | |
| Maintenance of anonymity of healthcare workers in case of exposure | Employee should not disclose other members of staff personal information |
| Adherence to Care Quality Commission (CQC) regulations—have adequate policies in place, be knowledgeable in dealing with sharps' injuries and the first occupational department a staff member has to be referred to | |

## 18.5 Higher Risk Groups

Certain groups of individuals are more prone to carrying blood-borne pathogens and so their presence as patients could lead to a higher risk of exposure to healthcare workers. All healthcare workers providing direct clinical care to a high-risk patient will have access to the medical records making them aware of the possibility of being exposed to blood-borne diseases.

- Injecting drug users.
- Men who have sex with other men.
- Sex workers.
- Individuals with a history of blood-borne pathogens.
- Individuals with chronic active hepatitis or cirrhosis.
- Individuals with haemophilia.
- Individuals with iatrogenic immunosuppression or low CD4 count.
- Sexual partners or offspring from the above groups.

## 18.6 Protocol for a Healthcare Worker Exposed to High-Risk Blood Sample

1. Blood sampling to prove seroconversion.
2. Counselling by Occupational Health department with regard to statistics of seroconversion, support networks, provision of confidentiality and instructions on when it is possible to return to work.
3. Approach source patient for blood-borne virus testing.
4. For prophylaxis, if patient has a known history of:

   HIV post-exposure prophylaxis (PEP), up to 72 h post-exposure.
   HCV no prophylaxis.
   HBV check immune status of exposed person.
   review blood samples at 6 weeks, 3 months and 6 months
   give HB booster if needed.
   consider accelerated vaccination programme.

## 18.7 Protocol for a Healthcare Worker Exposed to a Low-Risk or Stale Blood Sample

1. Obtain HCW's baseline blood sample to prove seroconversion or absence of it.
2. For prophylaxis, if patient has a known history of:

HIV Seroconversion is infrequent following occupational exposure.
Consideration should be given to baseline blood sample as number 1 above
HCV no prophylaxis
HBV check immune status of exposed person
review blood samples at 6 weeks, 3 months and 6 months
give booster given if needed
consider accelerated vaccination programme

## 18.8 Immediate Management of a Sharps Injury

The immediate approach that needs to be taken in case of a sharps injury involving blood-borne viruses is illustrated in Fig. 18.1.

Body fluid exposure incident

⇩

First aid
(splash eyes and mouth with water)

⇩

In case of injury to skin

- wash site immediately with water
- do NOT scrub injured area and do not use antiseptics
- gently encourage puncture wounds to bleed
- do NOT suck

⇩

Inform line manager

⇩

Fill in a clinical incident report on Datix®
(software program used which might vary between trusts)

⇩

Document all details of the patient and details of the incident

⇩

Fill in Patient Risk Assessment Form (PRAF)

⇩

Consent patient and healthcare worker for serological tests
If No consent is obtained seek advice from on-call consultant in the Infectious Disease Department

⇩

Inform the Health and Safety Officer and the Consultant in Occupational Health

If out-of-hours, contact the Consultant in A&E quoting the Datix®reference number

**Fig. 18.1** Flow diagram for management protocol in cases of blood-borne virus exposure

## 18.9 Occupational Health Service Management of a Needlestick Injury

The management of Occupational Health for healthcare professionals involved in needlestick is completed over a series of stages and involves both nursing and medical professionals. The process has been simplified in the form of a flow diagram illustrated in Fig. 18.2.

Assess the HCW immediately and determine if a significant injury has occurred.

⇩

Review the completed source patient BBV risk assessment form and if required discuss the results with the clinician looking after the source patient.

⇩

Undertake a risk assessment of the incident including an assessment of the injury and an assessment of the risk from the source patient and decide on appropriate action.

⇩

Arrange for bloods to be taken from the injured HCW for storage (if commencing PEP also baseline bloods for FBC, U&E's, LFT's, Lipids and Glucose.

⇩

Assess the need for HIV PEP, HBV vaccination and hepatitis B immunoglobulin.

⇩

Consult with the Infectious Disease physician on call if prescribing PEP or are unsure if PEP is indicated.

⇩

Administer PEP/ HBV vaccination/hep b immunoglobulin as required based on risk assessment.

⇩

Arrange follow up for BBV testing as required based on the risk assessment. (Follow up testing comprises of HIV at 6 and 12 weeks, HBV and HCV and 6,12 and 24 weeks).

⇩

Receive the anonymised result of the source patient BBV testing and report the results to the injured HCW.

⇩

Review the need for PEP/ HBV immunisation and follow up for BBV testing based on the source patient BBV test results if and when available.

⇩

If necessary, offer referral for specialist advice and support and arrange follow up with the Infectious Disease Physician if HIV PEP is started.

⇩

- Notify Health and Safety if an employee is injured by a sharp known to be contaminated with a blood borne virus and where an employee who sustains a high risk needlestick injury subsequently develops a BBV.

⇩

Notify the line manager of the employee's time off-work and planned date of return to work.

**Fig. 18.2** Flow diagram outlining Occupational health service management protocol for cases involving blood-borne viruses exposures

## 18.10 Legislation and Typical Trust Policies

Relevant trust policies and relevant legislations that would offer a systematic approach and further information, respectively to this situation are listed below in alphabetical order (the nomenclature of these policies varies between different trusts):

Policies:

- Inoculation Injury Policy.
- Prevention and Management of Needlestick and Sharps Injuries Policy.

Legislations and Standards:

- Control of Substances Hazardous to Health Regulations 2002 (COSHH).
- Health and Safety at Work 1974.
- Management of Health and Safety at Work Regulations 1999.
- Reporting of Injuries, Diseases and Dangerous Occurrences Regulations 1995 (RIDDOR).

## Further Reading

Department of Health (2008) HIV Post-Exposure Prophylaxis: Guidance from the UK Chief Medical Officers' Expert Advisory Group on AIDS, September 2008. https://assets.publishing.service.gov.uk/government/uploads/system/uploads/attachment_data/file/203139/HIV_post-exposure_prophylaxis.pdf. Accessed Jan 2020

Department of Health (2013) Recommendation for HIV post-exposure prophylaxis (PEP) following occupational exposure to a source with undetectable HIV viral load, December 2013. https://assets.publishing.service.gov.uk/government/uploads/system/uploads/attachment_data/file/275060/EAGA_advice_on_PEP_after_exposure_to_UD_source_Dec13.pdf. Accessed Jan 2020

Department of Health (2014) Change to recommended regimen for post-exposure prophylaxis (PEP), September 2014. https://assets.publishing.service.gov.uk/government/uploads/system/uploads/attachment_data/file/351633/Change_to_recommended_regimen_for_PEP_starter_pack_final.pdf. Accessed Jan 2020

# Management of Staff with Repeated Episodes of Absenteeism

# 19

**Scenario**

You are one of four consultants of a medical department in a UK teaching hospital.

The receptionists' line manager has just informed you that one of the receptionists whom you have not seen for a while is off again. The staff bank had to be contacted for an emergency replacement in order to cover the front desk of the department.

What do you do?

## 19.1 Introduction

When presented with this scenario, you will need to be able to discuss and expand on the following:

- Knowledge of employer regulations and entitlement to annual leave days.
- Knowledge of the process of requesting leave.
- Maternity leave, emergency leave and sick leave.

## 19.2 Main Types of Leave Entitlements

The following is a list of the main types of leave entitlements in alphabetical order:

1. Annual leave
2. Carer's Leave
3. Compassionate or Bereavement Leave
4. Emergency leave
5. Jury Service Leave



S. Abela, *Leadership and Management in Healthcare*,
https://doi.org/10.1007/978-3-031-21025-9_19

6. Maternity leave
7. Parental leave
8. Paternity leave
9. Professional leave
10. Sickness leave
11. Special leave
12. Study leave
13. Trade Union Duties Leave

### 19.2.1 Maternity Leave

All NHS employees who are pregnant regardless of the position, length of work or the number of hours contracted to work are entitled to maternity leave and allowances.

Below are the types of maternity pays and allowances:

- Statutory maternity leave (SML)
- Statutory maternity pay (SMP)
- Ordinary maternity leave (OML)
- Occupational maternity pay (OMP)
- Maternity allowance (MA)
- Additional maternity leave (AML)

**Statutory Maternity Leave (SML)**

Eligible employees, who have worked with their employer continuously for at least 26 weeks into the 'qualifying week' (the 15th week before the expected week of childbirth), can take up to 52 weeks' maternity leave. The first 26 weeks is known as 'Ordinary Maternity Leave' (OML), the last 26 weeks as 'Additional Maternity Leave' (AML).

The earliest that leave can be taken is 11 weeks before the expected week of childbirth, unless the baby is born early.

Employees must take at least 2 weeks after the birth.

**Statutory Maternity Pay (SMP)**

SMP for eligible employees can be paid for up to 39 weeks, usually as follows:

- The first 6 weeks: 90% of their average weekly earnings (AWE) before tax.
- The remaining 33 weeks: £145.18 or 90% of their average weekly earnings [AWE (whichever is lower)]

**Maternity Allowance (MA)**

MA is granted when an employee is not entitled to SMP but meets qualifying conditions based on their recent employment and earnings records. This entitlement's maximum is of 39 weeks.

MA is paid at the same weekly rate as the standard rate of SMP, throughout the MA period. The main difference between MA and SMP is the higher rate for the first 6 weeks.

Employees must have been employed or self-employed for at least 26 weeks of the 66-week period up to the beginning of the expected week of childbirth.

Earnings must be £30 per week or more over a 13-week period. MA can start as early as 11 weeks prior to childbirth and the latest is 1 day following birth. Failure to return to work does not necessitate repayment of the MA received.

Maternity allowances are based on two factors:

1. Intention to return to work.
2. Service provision for the NHS (in weeks or years). Figures 19.1, 19.2 and 19.3 provide the maternity allowances for staff that have been in post for less than 26 weeks, between 26 and 52 weeks and more than 52 weeks respectively.

**Occupational Maternity Pay (OMP)**

OMP is an optional payment that the employer pays in addition to the SMP.

OMP is usually reserved for employees that return to work after childbirth.

The employee's SMP entitlement is governed by the Department for Works and Pensions, however, the OMP's entitlement is defined by the employer and acts as an incentive for the employee to return to work following childbirth or not change a company by increasing loyalty.

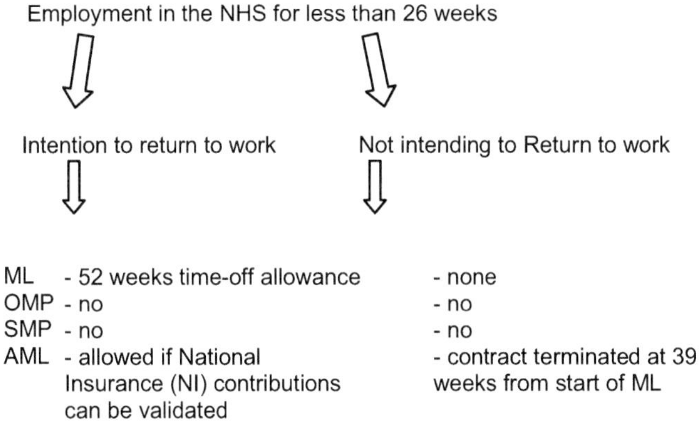


**Fig. 19.1** Flow diagram for staff requesting maternity leave and have been employed with the NHS for less than 26 weeks

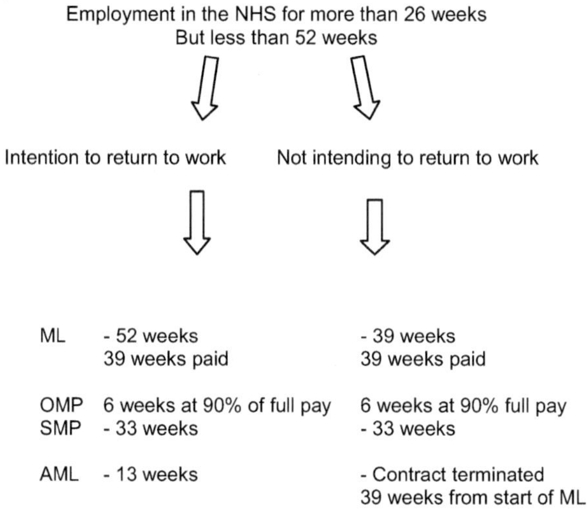


**Fig. 19.2** Flow diagram for staff requesting maternity leave and employed with the NHS for more than 26 weeks but less than 52 weeks

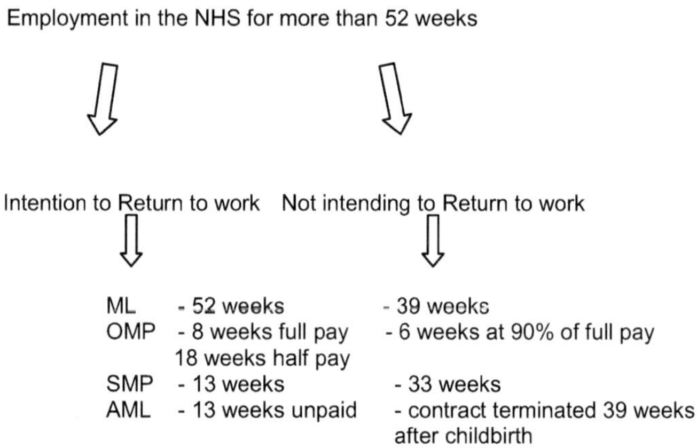


**Fig. 19.3** Flow diagram for staff requesting maternity leave and employed with the NHS for more than 52 weeks

## Employer and Employees' Responsibilities during Maternity Period

The following checklists outline the duties of both the employer via the line manager and the employee once the pregnancy is confirmed:

Manager's Checklist:

As soon as employee advises you of pregnancy:

- Carry out a risk assessment exercise to ascertain safety at work.
- Allow paid time off for all medical antenatal appointments.

Once written confirmation of maternity leave is received from an employee:

- Acknowledge receipt of maternity information from employee within 28 days.
- Confirm the possibility of a flexible return to work; part-time or full-time.
- Plan staff cover during the employee's absence period.
- Confirm accrual and remainder of annual leave and discuss when to take it.
- Complete the trust's maternity form and a leaver's form—ESR3.
- Discuss visits or 'Keeping in Touch' days if appropriate.

Before employee returns to work:

- Consider any requests for flexible working.
- Consider possible arrangements for breastfeeding.
- Give formal notice to any temporary staff covering this area of work—temporary employment terms would have been specified by the human resources department at the recruitment stage.

Employee's Checklist:
At the confirmation stage by the employee:

- Write to the line manager by the 15th week before baby is due.
- Give at least 28 days' notice of any change to the start of maternity leave.
- Give 8 weeks' notice of any change to the date of return from maternity leave.
- Discuss your return and any additional needs with the manager.
- Discuss any unused annual leave.
- Present the trust's maternity form and sign and return promptly.
- Discuss visits or 'Keeping in Touch' days if appropriate.

Before returning:

- Agree arrangements for returning to work, including any request for flexible working.
- Advise whether breastfeeding arrangements are required.

### 19.2.2 Paternity Leave

When requested, the maximum duration of paternity leave is 2 weeks following the baby's birth. This could be taken in one block of 2 weeks or two separate blocks of 1 week each. If the baby is born prematurely the paternity leave should be taken up to 8 weeks following the baby's birth.

PL allowance is usually granted at the 15th week before childbirth however like ML, it is also related to the previous employment with the NHS.

Cancellation of the paternity leave needs a 28 days' notice.

Statutory paternity pay and pay are granted following the completion of an SC3 form or SC4. The former is for employees who will become birth parents and the latter is for employees who will be adopting a child.

Table 19.1 tabulates the PL allowance for the two types of PL.

SPP is £145.18 per week and if earnings are less than £116 per week then SPP is calculated at 90% of the staff member's weekly earnings.

If earnings are less than National Lower Earnings Limit (NLEL); £107, then an application for Income support during paternity leave is supported.

These figures are subject to change following parliamentary changes.

**Parental Leave (PRL)**

PRL gives parents the chance to take a period of time off work to look after a child. This leave can also be claimed by parents who adopt a child.

PRL is usually 18 weeks, four of which are paid and the remainder unpaid unless an individual agreement has been set up between the employer and employee.

The paid part of this leave can be claimed up to the child's 14th birthday whilst the unpaid part of this leave can be taken up to 18 weeks prior to the child's 18th birthday.

Trusts usually prefer if PRL is taken in blocks or multiples of 1 week (Fig. 19.4).

**Table 19.1** Paternity leave allowance

| Type of allowance | <26 weeks of employment | >26 but <52 weeks of employment | >52 weeks of employment |
|---|---|---|---|
| PL | 2 weeks | 2 weeks | 2 weeks |
| OPL (ordinary paternity pay) | No | No | Yes |
| SPP (statutory paternal pay) | No | Yes | Yes |

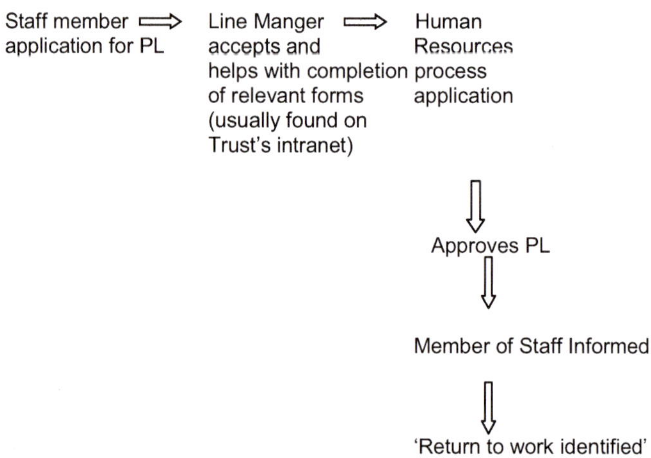


**Fig. 19.4** Process of PL application

**Table 19.2** SL entitlement based on history of previous employment

| Employment history with the NHS | Full-pay in months | Half-pay in months |
|---|---|---|
| More than 6 years | 6 | 6 |
| Between 4 and 5 years | 5 | 5 |
| 3 years | 4 | 4 |
| 2 years | 2 | 2 |
| 1 year | 1 | 1 |

### Sickness Leave (SL)

Generally, an employer accepts a self-certified sick leave of less than 7 days, however, a 'fit note' is needed if SL is more than 7 days. This is usually obtained from a certified general practitioner.

The amount of SL entitled is dependent on the length of the employee's placement history in the post. Table 19.2 aims to simplify this type of entitlement.

Once the full entitlement of SL is surpassed, statutory sick pay (SSP) is granted. This amounts to £92.05 per week and it is paid by the employer for up to 28 weeks.

### Study Leave

Study leave entitlement applies for both full and part-time trainees. The maximum number of days study leave per year is 30 days for a full-time trainee whilst a part-time trainee would have this calculated pro-rata. The trainee can liaise with the Training Programme Director (TPD) to establish an accurate figure and can also ask for 7 of these days to be prepared for an official examination.

The allocated funding to subsidise the studies for a full-time trainee is £805. This is also calculated pro-rata for a part-time trainee and the budget is allocated between March and the end of February each year.

Neither the study leave nor the study leave budget are transferrable from 1 year to another.

Any leave applications are made through the study leave administrators and approved by the TPD. All pertinent receipts should be submitted with the application form and processed before a cut-off date stipulated by the administrators. Rail travel is reimbursed at second-class rate and car travel is reimbursed at 23 pence per mile travelled. Accommodation is subsidised at £55 per night and sustenance at £20 per day.

### Professional Leave (PL)

Professional leave refers to other or additional entitlement of time off work aside from that granted for courses.

PL can be used for research, teaching, examining or taking examinations, visiting clinics and attending professional conferences. PL is not only limited to trainees but also to NHS staff once the necessary approval is obtained by the relevant line managers.

Below is a list of all the duties that can be covered by PL:

- Duties as an officer, an assessor or as a committee member or member of a working party of a Royal College, Faculty, Professional or Scientific Society or NICE.
  - Examining commitments or a regional advisor role for the Royal Colleges, Universities or other related institutions.
  - Attendance for work-related activities for the Department of Health.
  - Duties as a member of a Mental Health Act Commission.
  - Duties as a member of a Medical Defence Society.
  - Attendance at British or International Standards Committees.
  - Duties as a member of the Medical Research Council.
  - Membership of the Editorial Board of a Scientific Journal.
  - Duties in relation to postgraduate educational activities outside the Trust.
  - Lecturing commitments.
  - Visits to hospitals outside the Region for the purpose of assessing training facilities
- Undergraduate or postgraduate lectures.

PL is granted at the discretion of the organisation for which the employee is working. This is also the case for any monetary funds applied to cover the expenses associated with the proposed activity.

**Emergency Leave (EL)**

NHS Employees may be able to take 1 or 2 days of paid leave at short notice to deal with emergency circumstances. If more leave is required this may be granted at the discretion of the manager as annual leave or unpaid leave.

Emergency leave is intended for urgent situations that could not be foreseen. It usually involves looking after dependents. Other unforeseen circumstances include the following:

- If a dependent has been involved in an accident.
- A dependent who suffers from a long-term illness.
- Emergency child care during school hours.
- Urgent domestic situations such as fire, flood or burglary.

**Amount of EL**

Normally, 1 day is permitted, however, time off can be extended in case this is needed to deal with an urgent situation.

This could be permitted by the line manager as unplanned annual leave or unpaid leave. The maximum entitled EL is up to 22.5 h paid leave that may be given in any rolling 12-month period which is calculated pro rata for part-time employees. There is no right to paid emergency leave.

In exceptional circumstances, a request for extended special leave may be made to a senior manager. Up to 3 months of unpaid leave may be granted as special leave or combined with annual leave. Requests for a longer period may be considered under the Employment Break Scheme/Policy or Career Break Policy.

**Management of EL**

Due to the urgent nature of the matters necessitating EL, the decision on the employee's funding allowance will be confirmed on the employee's return. The employee's line manager and the Human Resources department would log the number of days off for the employee and confirm the allowance unless a decision has not already been made.

**Bereavement Leave (BL)**

Bereavement Leave is the granting of leave on compassionate grounds. This type of leave can also be referred to as Compassionate Leave. The leave entitlement may be available to all employees regardless of the length of employment, although the time off may vary depending on whether the deceased is an immediate family member or more distant. In the event of a death involving an immediate relative (normally defined as a spouse, civil partner, child, parent or sibling of the employee) 1–2 days of paid special leave may be granted. This allows enough time to make all the necessary funeral arrangements. In exceptional circumstances a further 2 days paid special leave may be given (i.e. up to a maximum of 5 paid days in total).

If a death involves a close relative (normally defined as a grandparent, niece, nephew, aunt/uncle or immediate relative of a partner) up to 2 days of unpaid special leave may be granted.

Further time off may be granted at the discretion of the employee's line manager, which may be taken as annual or unpaid leave.

**Carer's Leave (CL)**

Employees who are also carers of adults who are disabled, ill or elderly can request unpaid carer's leave of up to 1 week per year. This leave is also subject to the following criteria:

- 1 year of continuous service with the NHS.
- 21 days' notice unless there is an urgent need, in writing.

Should the situation be a recurring one with an impact on the working hours or other team members, the employee might want to request short-term flexibility. This request will be subject to the manager's discretion and dependent on the service requirements.

If the agreed flexibility is for less than 1 month and the hours worked are staying the same, the arrangement will be informal.

For longer periods of time and where hours will change, the employee is encouraged to follow the Flexible Working Policy and Procedure to apply for a change of hours.

**Jury Service Leave**

Jury Service is compulsory in the UK. Jurors are selected at random from the electoral roll. An employee who received a jury summons is expected to attend.

Employees will automatically be granted paid time off work unless they are claiming expenses from the courts for loss of earnings. In exceptional circumstances, the line manager might request a postponement of jury service due to demands on the service. This process is initiated by filling the summons for jury service form; approval of this postponement will be the court's decision. A second postponement, is not usually possible.

Procedure

When an employee receives a summon for jury service form they should discuss the request with their manager.

**Trade Union Leave**

An employee who is officially affiliated with a Trade Union will be allowed reasonable time off with pay during working hours to carry out union duties or undergo training for union duties.

Trusts would have a policy for Trade Union Duties and Activities.

## 19.3 Management of Colleagues with Repeated Episodes of Absenteeism

In cases where a colleague displays patterns of abnormal sickness leave or is repeatedly absent from work for unknown reasons, a sequential approach should be followed, such as the one suggested below:

1. Observe abnormal patterns.
2. Alert the colleague's relevant line manager.
3. Investigate appropriately and substantiate observed patterns.
   - Is this a one-off episode or has it happened multiple times?
   - Is support needed?
4. The Human Resources (HR) department should be informed.
5. HR measures absenteeism and identifies the 'Emerging Pattern'.
6. Bradford Sickness Score (BSS) should be measured. This is based on the formula:

$$B = S^2 \times D$$

Key:

*B* Bradford score.

*S* Sickness score (the resultant score after adding the multiplication of the number of episodes of sickness with the number of sick days claimed).

*D* Number of sick days (the addition of all the sick days claimed).

BSS is based on the fact that multiple single episodes of sick leave cause more disruption than single longer spells. HR calculates BSS over a period of 52 weeks or 12 months. A score of higher than 128 or more than 3 episodes every 6 months should trigger investigative procedures.

Below is a worked example:

An employee has been reported sick 5 times each time being off duty for 5 days and amounting to 25 days.

Sickness score: 1(5) + 1(5) + 1(5) + 1(5) + 1(5) = 5

Number of sick 5 + 5 + 5 + 5 + 5 = 25 days

Formula: $B = S^2 \times D$
Calculation: $B = 5^2 \times 25$
Bradford score: 625

Please note that this score would be considered very high.

Figure 19.5 illustrates a stepwise approach for the management of a member of staff with repeated episodes of reported absences due to sickness.

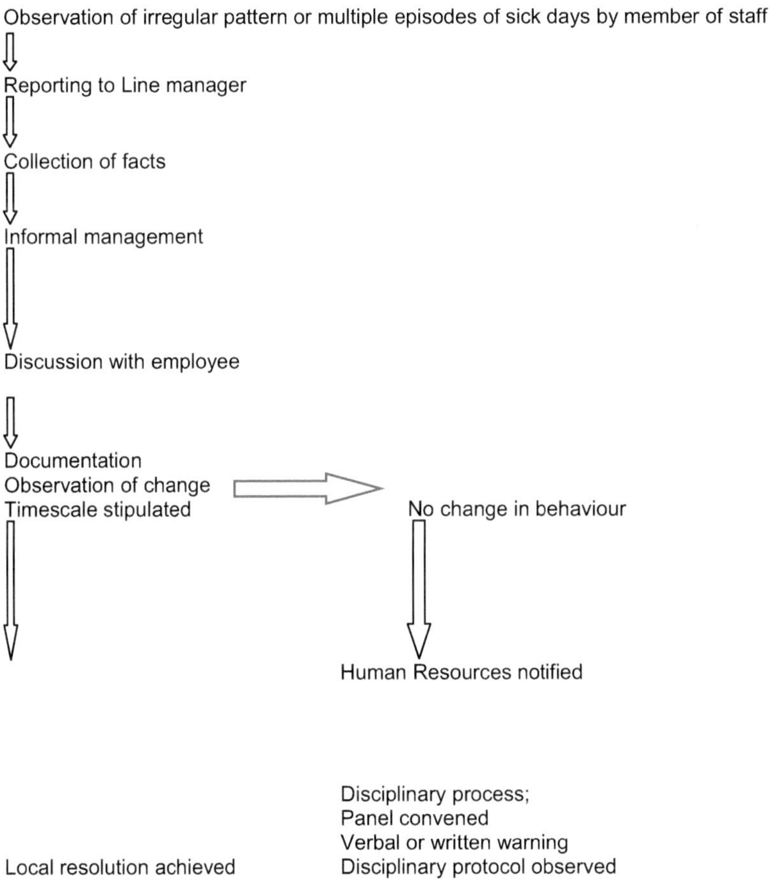


**Fig. 19.5** Flow diagram illustrating the management of this scenario

## 19.4 Typical Trust Policies

Relevant trust policies and relevant legislations that would offer a systematic approach and further information, respectively, to this situation are listed below in alphabetical order (the nomenclature of these policies varies between different trusts):

- Annual Leave Calculator Guidelines
- Career Break
- Managing Sickness Absence
- Maternity Leave
- Parental Leave
- Special Leave

# Management of a New Business Case 20

> **Scenario**
> You are a consultant in a district general hospital.
> You are asked by your management team to make 2.5% savings. You have also identified the need for a new part-time clinician at a staff grade level.
> What do you do?

## 20.1 Introduction

Every NHS organisation will have its individual business case templates and documents which might vary between different organisations. These templates and documents are also regularly modified and updated in line with the respective standing financial instructions.

In general, the process of a business case approval will vary depending on the following factors:

1. Budget allocation for the proposal.
2. Expenditure type: Capital or Revenue.
3. Pay or non-pay type of proposal.
4. Value of business case.
5. Long-term use of business case proposal.

The first step to assessing the financial position of a department is to undertake a financial analysis. Income generation should be directly compared to the expenditure and aspects or services generating profit or loss should be identified. Profit can be increased by either increasing the revenue or by cost-cutting exercises.



S. Abela, *Leadership and Management in Healthcare*,
https://doi.org/10.1007/978-3-031-21025-9_20

When presented with this scenario you will need to be able to discuss and expand on the following:

- Recognise areas where savings can be made.
- Knowledge of how to implement savings.
- Knowledge of how to apply for funding for recruitment of new staff.
- Knowledge of recruitment process once a new post is approved.

## 20.2 Business Cases

Generally, the process of preparing for a new business case proposal involves five key stages and the business case application then usually comprises four main sections. In this scenario, the application is for a new member of staff to join your department. The same principles apply to an application for new equipment or other requirements.

Five key stages in a new business case proposal:

1. Identify the need for a new [member of staff].
2. Identify the trust's hospital pro forma (this form varies between trusts and it is usually available on the trust's intranet).
3. Discuss the benefits of the proposed investment with the appropriate stakeholders including head of department, line managers, clinical director and head of directorate.
4. Present the business case and gain approval from the Clinical Effectiveness Committee (nomenclature and committee structures vary between trusts).
5. Obtain approval of the business case by the Clinical Governance Committee (nomenclature and committee structures vary between trusts).

Main sections of a typical trust business case application

1. Executive Summary
   Outline the need for a new member of staff. For each business case the summary would have three subsections to highlight the advantages, in this scenario, of a new member of staff, listed below:
   (a) Income generation
   (b) For specialist/higher training
   (c) Succession planning
2. Background Information
   Outline the most important aspects of your service:
   (a) Structure of the department
   (b) Type of conditions patients present with
   (c) The training doctors are involved in
   (d) The teaching activity
   (e) The research performance

3. Proposal
   Outline your proposal and any other potential options in order to give the committees the chance to opt for the best option.
   The strengths and weaknesses of each proposal have to be discussed.
4. Income generation versus expenditure
   Here you have to demonstrate that the additional expenditure (on a new member of staff) will result in a financial gain, through extra income generation.

## 20.3 Management of Applying for a New Member of Staff

When proposing additions to the existing workforce, trust committees look at the additional income generated with the increased activity brought about by the new member of staff.

In this scenario, you might be able to demonstrate that the increased activity and income generation by the department as a result of employing a new member of staff is equivalent to a budget saving of 2.5%.

No matter what percentage of savings is required by the trust's management, the process always starts by obtaining a budget sheet.

Figure 20.1 is an example of a typical budget sheet for an operational department within an NHS trust.

| Accounts for Department 1 in DGH 2 [Month 3] | | | | | | | | | | |
|---|---|---|---|---|---|---|---|---|---|---|
| CURRENT BUDGET (WTE) | Current contract (WTE) | Account code | Description | Current year budget | Current period budget | Current period expenditure | Current period variance | Current budget to date | Cumulative expenditure to date | Cumulative variance to date |
| | | 1 | Consultant | | | | | | | |
| | | 12 | Associate Specialist | | | | | | | |
| | | 13 | Staff Practitioner | | | | | | | |
| | | 14 | Hospital Practitioner | | | | | | | |
| | | 15 | ST Trainees (Deanery Funded) | | | | | | | |
| | | 16 | Locum Consultant | | | | | | | |
| | | 17 | Locum Grade Doctor | | | | | | | |
| | | 18 | Locum SpR | | | | | | | |
| | | 19 | Specialty QPP | | | | | | | |
| | | 20 | Medical Practitioner | | | | | | | |
| | | | Pay Expenditure | | | | | | | |
| | | | | | | | | | | |
| | | 100 | Teaveling and Substinstence | | | | | | | |
| | | 101 | Stationery | | | | | | | |
| | | 102 | Advertising | | | | | | | |
| | | | | | | | | | | |
| | | 200 | Interview Expenses | | | | | | | |
| | | 201 | Training | | | | | | | |
| | | 202 | Specialty Qipp Non-Pay | | | | | | | |
| | | | Non-Expenditure Pay | | | | | | | |
| | | | | | | | | | | |
| | | 300 | Non-staff Recharge Pay | | | | | | | |
| | | | Income | | | | | | | |
| | | | | | | | | | | |
| | | | Total for Department | | | | | | | |

**Fig. 20.1** An example of a typical budget sheet for a department within a Trust

It usually consists of two main parts:

1. Pay-related items which is mainly constituted by staff salaries.
2. Non-pay related items such as consumables, equipment and stationery items amongst others.

The pay-related items are usually the biggest expenditure of the department and this invariably equates to approximately 65% of the whole department's budget.

Each budget is measured per financial year which spans from April to April. The trusts' accountants thus refer to April as month 1 of the budget year. Every trust operates with the same financial calendar, with April being the first month of every financial year.

Figure 20.2 shows a typical monthly budget sheet of a department within an NHS trust.

Key:

Actual: The current expenditure.
Budget: The projected expenditure in advance.
Variance: The total difference between the actual expenditure and that projected at the start of the year.

Taking the hypothetical department's budget sheet for month 3 of the year shown above, the total expenditure is budgeted to be £405,400. The management has asked for savings of 2.5% which is approximately £10,000.

**Accounts for Department 1 in DGH 2 [Month 3]**

| CURRENT BUDGET (WTE) | Current contract (WTE) | Account code | Description | Current year budget | Current period budget | Current period expenditure | Current period variance | Current budget to date | Cumulative expenditure to date | Cumulative variance to date |
|---|---|---|---|---|---|---|---|---|---|---|
| 1.5 | 0.55 | 1 | Consultant | 251,000 | 20,917 | 4,242 | −16675 | 146,417 | 34,816 | −111601 |
| 0.18 | 0.18 | 12 | Associate Specialist | 17,200 | 1433 | 1,284 | −149 | 10,033 | 8,988 | −1045 |
| 0.09 | 0 | 13 | Staff Practitioner | 6,000 | 500 | 0 | −500 | 3,500 | 0 | −3500 |
| 0.59 | 0.14 | 14 | Hospital Practitioner | 49,300 | 4,108 | 809 | −3299 | 28,758 | 5,665 | −23093 |
| 2 | 2 | 15 | ST Trainees (Deanery Funded) | 91,200 | 7,700 | 7,697 | −3 | 52,700 | 52,199 | −501 |
| 0 | 0 | 16 | Locum Consultant | 0 | 0 | 0 | 0 | 0 | 43,852 | 43,852 |
| 0 | 0.2 | 17 | Locum Grade Doctor | 200 | 17 | 1,287 | 1,270 | 117 | 9,007 | 8,890 |
| 0 | 0 | 18 | Locum SpR | 0 | 0 | 0 | 0 | 0 | −102 | −102 |
| 0 | 0 | 19 | Specialty QPP | −3600 | −300 | 0 | 300 | −2100 | 0 | 2,100 |
| 0.09 | 0.09 | 20 | Medical Practitioner | 6000 | 500 | 395 | −105 | 3,500 | 2,768 | −732 |
| **4.45** | **3.16** | | **Pay Expenditure** | **417,300** | **34,875** | **15,714** | **19,161** | **242,925** | **157,193** | **−85732** |
| | | | | | | | | | | |
| 0 | 0 | 100 | Teaveling and Substinstence | 100 | 8 | 0 | −8 | 58 | 0 | −58 |
| 0 | 0 | 101 | Stationery | 5300 | 442 | 1832 | 1390 | 3,092 | 5495 | 2,404 |
| 0 | 0 | 102 | Advertising | 6100 | 508 | −253 | −761 | 3,558 | 4403 | 845 |
| 0 | 0 | 200 | Interview Expenses | 0 | 0 | 0 | 0 | 0 | 55 | 55 |
| 0 | 0 | 201 | Training | 0 | 0 | 0 | 0 | 0 | 340 | 340 |
| 0 | 0 | 202 | Speciality Qipp Non-Pay | −400 | −33 | 0 | 33 | −233 | 0 | 233 |
| 0 | 0 | | **Non-Expenditure Pay** | **11,100** | **925** | **1,579** | **654** | **6,475** | **10,293** | **3,818** |
| | | | | | | | | | | |
| 0 | 0 | 300 | Non-staff Recharge Pay | −23000 | −1917 | 0 | 1917 | −13417 | −11474 | 1943 |
| 0 | 0 | | **Income** | **−23000** | **−1917** | **0** | **1917** | **−13417** | **−11474** | **1943** |
| | | | | | | | | | | |
| **4.45** | **3.16** | | **Total for Department 1** | **405,400** | **33,883** | **17,294** | **−16590** | **235,983** | **156,013** | **−79971** |

**Fig. 20.2** A typical monthly budget sheet of a department within an NHS trust

With the knowledge of recruitment in due course, the advertising budget can be saved as no more advertisements will be placed. This will save a total of £61,000. In addition, a cut in the stationery expenditure can also be identified due to an existing surplus of stock. A saving of £3900 is identified as a realistic target out of the total yearly budget of £5300, leaving a budget of £1400 for stationary expenses, thus producing the requested saving.

The savings will also be supplemented by the income generated by the increased activity of the new member of staff. The activity income is measured by analysing the type of procedures being carried out and the amount of procedures per day. This will give the total income generated. The saving will be offset against the new team member's salary, however, the income generated will be a surplus for the department.

## 20.4 Main Sources of Income Generation and Savings within a Hospital Department

As mentioned earlier in this chapter, a financial analysis is necessary to identify areas or services within a department that could lead to greater profit by increasing revenue or by cost-cutting measures.

Income generation can be increased by:

- Increasing the number of referrals received.
- Increasing threshold of the number of referrals received by justifying it with the local commissioners.
- Ensuring the coding process is done correctly and in a timely manner.
- Provision of educational courses and training.
- Provision of private healthcare services.
- Set up payments for repairs of devices or loss of NHS's equipment.
- Research funding.
- Ensuring payments are upheld for overseas visitors seeking treatment.

Additional income streams can include charging for car parking, catering services, accommodation, advertising and temporary use of facilities and buildings.

Cost-cutting measures are ideally classified as pay or non-pay related.

Pay-related cost-cutting measures can include the following:

- Revision of staff numbers needed.
- Revision for the need of temporary or locum staff.
- Early retirement when appropriate.
- Actioning a freeze on jobs.
- Altering the staff profile and allowing a better skill mix.

Non-pay related cost-cutting measures can include the following:

- Consumable cuts.
- Altering the procurement sources for the consumables for cheaper alternatives.
- Off-site services comparison to on-site services such as manufacturing of devices.
- Outsourcing services that are cheaper such as cleaning, housekeeping and central sterilisation services.

## 20.5 Typical Trust Policies

Relevant trust policies that would offer a systematic approach and further information, respectively, to this situation are listed below in alphabetical order (the nomenclature of these policies varies between different trusts):

- New therapy and procedure policy
- Budget Management Policy
- Freedom of Information Policy
- Income Policy
- Standards for Business Conduct Policy
- Charitable Funds Policy

# Management of a Dilemma Involving Sharing of Confidential Information and Professional Conduct

# 21

> **Scenario**
>
> You are a year 5 (St5) surgical trainee and have been working in the same department for 9 months.
>
> A trainee colleague approaches you and confides that his recent blood tests were positive for HIV, a blood-borne virus. He does not want to disclose the information to anyone and wants his status to remain unknown.
>
> What do you do?

## 21.1 Introduction

When presented with this scenario you will need to be able to discuss and expand on the following:

- The management of HIV-infected healthcare workers.
- Knowledge of the government's documents.
- Knowledge of handling confidential information.
- Knowledge of hospital policies and occupational health protocols for HIV-infected medical professionals to treat patients.

## 21.2 Legal Obligations

It is the responsibility of the healthcare worker together with the Trust employing the latter, to protect the health and safety of the patients. It is the Trusts' responsibility to safeguard the confidential health status of the employee whilst ensuring that they get a fair and just employment as any other employee employed by the



S. Abela, *Leadership and Management in Healthcare*,
https://doi.org/10.1007/978-3-031-21025-9_21

respective trust. The trust must also ensure that no risk is posed to the patients or other members of staff by the employed members who are positive for HIV.

The employee is legally obliged to disclose the health status if performance includes EPPs—Exposure Prone Procedures.

Employees have a right to receive any form of support whilst maintaining confidentiality and this is usually coordinated via the Occupational Health Service.

## 21.3 Management of a Colleague with a Blood-Borne Virus

Figure 21.1 shows a simplified protocol for management of HIV-infected Healthcare Workers (HCWs). The information has been reproduced from the DoH document: 'The Management of HIV-infected Healthcare Workers', a report produced by the tripartite working group, April 2011. Access to this document can be readily achieved via:

https://assets.publishing.service.gov.uk/government/uploads/system/uploads/attachment_data/file/216126/dh_131574.pdf—accessed March 2020.

This publication has been withdrawn and the current guidance is published by Public Heath England, accessible via: https://assets.publishing.service.gov.uk/government/uploads/system/uploads/attachment_data/file/909553/Integrated_guidance_for_management_of_BBV_in_HCW.pdf.—accessed March 2021.

The guidance has been last updated in August 2020 and is entitled; 'Integrated guidance on health clearance and the management of HCWs living with BBVs (hepatitis B, hepatitis C and HIV)'. A quick reference guide is also available.

All infected HCWs should meet the following criteria to be allowed to perform exposure-prone procedures (EEP):

- Be on combination antiretroviral therapy (cART) and have a plasma viral load of less than 200 copies per millilitre (<200 copies/ml).
- Be able to control and limit viral load below limes of assay detection for at least 12 months on three separate blood tests, referred to as 'elite controllers'.

Elite controllers have to have plasma load monitoring every 3 months, be under a Consultant in Occupational Therapy and be registered on UKAP Occupational Health Monitoring Register (UKAP-OHR).

Key:

| | |
|---|---|
| cART | Combination Anti-retroviral Therapy |
| EEP | Exposure-prone procedures |
| HCW | Healthcare Worker |
| HIV | Human Immunodeficiency Virus |
| OH | Occupational Health |
| RA | Risk Assessment |
| UKAP | United Kingdom Advisory Panel |
| VL | Viral Load |

**Fig. 21.1** A practical approach to clearance

| **HIV-positive HCWs initially cleared**<br>HCWs should be on cART | |
|---|---|
| VL test result:<br>< 200 copies/ml | - A case-by-case approach is needed<br>- A viral load of less than 200 copies on 2 different occasions no less than 3 months apart<br>- UKAP-OHR should be notified before clearance is granted |
| | |
| **On-going monitoring of HIV positive HCWs following health clearance** | |
| VL counted test result: | |
| < 50 copies/ml or below | No action- retest in 3 months |
| 50-200 copies/ml | -A case-by-case approach is needed<br>-Consider retaking blood sample in 10 days<br>-Consider limiting HCW's activity |
| >200 copies/ml | -Retake blood sample<br>-if VL is verified >200 copies/ml cease EPP activities<br>-Return to full practice if VL is <200 copies/ml on 2 consecutive tests less than 3 months apart |
| >1000 copies/ml | -All EPPs stopped<br>-Retake blood sample 10 days later to verify result<br>-If VL >1000 copies/ml is verified carry out RA and patient cross-matching<br>-Consider Patient Notification Exercise (PNE) based on RA<br>-HCW are required to keep a log of patients treated |
| | |
| **HCW not cleared – All EPPs ceased**<br>Pursue: i) RA - risk assessment exercise<br>ii) PNE - patient notification exercise | |

## 21.4 Management of Scenario

Possession of key information and knowledge is needed to manage the scenario presented in this chapter. The following are healthcare obligations that need to be followed and applied in scenarios involving sharing of confidential information.

- It is not a legal requirement to inform your employer about your HIV status, however, it is a legal obligation to do so for healthcare workers involved with exposure-prone procedures. This includes all surgical specialties including dental surgery.
- Disclosure should be made confidentially with no compromises on your post as it is not permitted for an employee to be shown discrimination by his or her employer. HIV is protected as a disability under the 2010 Equality Act.
- A hospital or other healthcare providers may share medical information including HIV status with another NHS provider, with the employee's permission.
- Every employee has the right to access the trust's occupational health department or the counselling services.
- With the exception of those involved with the exposure-prone procedures, disclosure is the employee's choice. The trust should offer support for disclosure followed by all the psychological and medical support needed to overcome all the consequences of the medial concealment.

This scenario provides a conflicting situation for any medical professional due to the responsibilities that a doctor's profession entails; confidentiality and patients' safety. The clinicians involved in scenarios such as the one described above, need to also be aware of the following key facts:

- Upon disclosure, the confidante has concealed his/her medical history which is confidential and should only be shared with his or her permission.
- Patients' safety is of prime concern and this disclosure must be reported if the individual concerned is involved with exposure-prone procedures.
- The first step is to listen to your colleague and ascertain factual information. Discuss the possibility of false positive results and that he or she might want to request a repeat test.
- Offer support and any cover as needed with authorisation from the clinical lead.
- Inform the individual about the counselling services that the trust offers and encourage them to reveal their medical history to the relevant medical officers.
- Reassuring him or her of confidentiality of their medical condition.
- Obtain permission from the individual to discuss the situation with experts and senior members of staff.

- If there are no further concerns, continue to offer any personal support you might be able to offer.
- If concerns persist, discuss the matters with your Indemnity society.
- If the trainee is providing EPP and there are concerns about patients' safety, the department's lead and the trust's occupational department must be informed.

Figure 21.2 illustrates a stepwise approach to managing cases involving disclosure of confidential information.

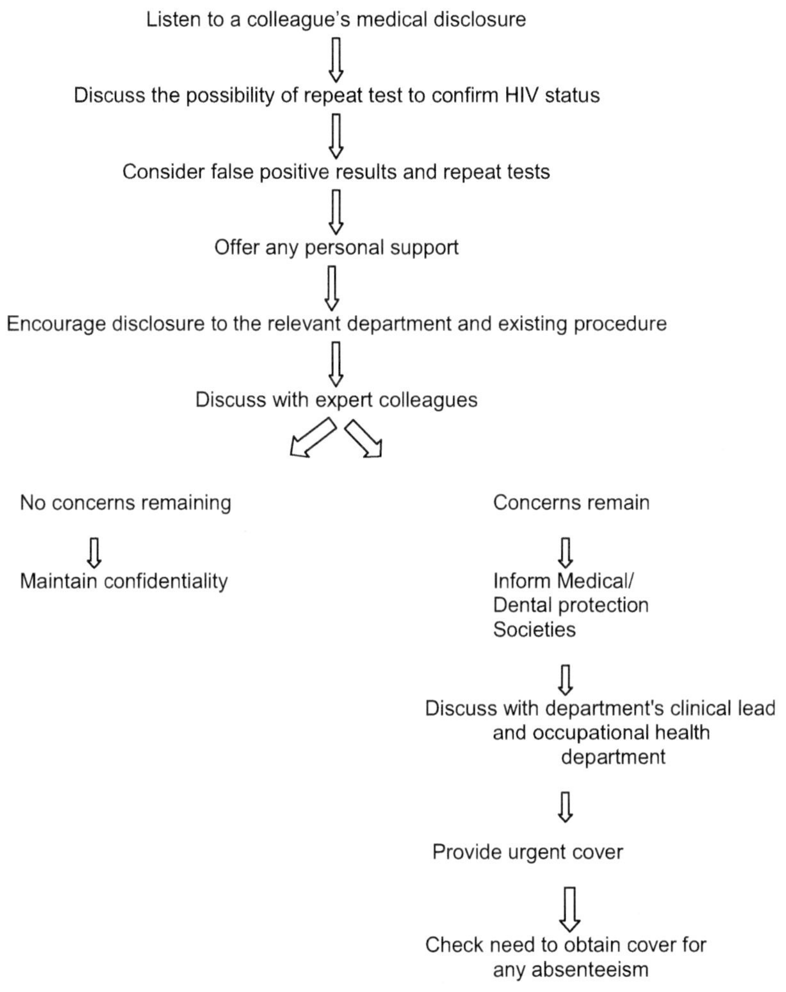


**Fig. 21.2** Typical management steps in cases involving disclosure of confidential information

## 21.5 Guidances, Legislations and Typical Trust Policies

Legislations:

- Equality Act 2010

Guidances:

- Public Health England (2020) Integrated guidance on health clearance of healthcare workers and the management of healthcare workers living with bloodborne viruses (hepatitis B, hepatitis C and HIV); Guidance from the UK Advisory Panel for Healthcare Workers Infected with Bloodborne Viruses (UKAP).
  [https://assets.publishing.service.gov.uk/government/uploads/system/uploads/attachment_data/file/909553/Integrated_guidance_for_management_of_BBV_in_HCW.pdf—accessed March 2021].
- Public Health England (2020) Integrated guidance on health clearance of healthcare workers and the management of healthcare workers living with bloodborne viruses (hepatitis B, hepatitis C and HIV): a quick reference guide, August 2020.
  [https://assets.publishing.service.gov.uk/government/uploads/system/uploads/attachment_data/file/908746/Integrated_guidance_on_BBV_in_HCW_v2.1_Quick_reference_guide_updated_August_2020.pdf—accessed March 2021].

Relevant trust policies that would offer a systematic approach and further information, respectively, to this situation are listed below in alphabetical order (the nomenclature of these policies varies between different trusts):

Policies:

- Code of Conduct Policy.
- Data Protection and Confidentiality Policy.
- Speak-out Policy.
- Management of HIV and AIDS Infected Healthcare Workers Policy.

# 22 Management of a Non-compliant Trainee

> **Scenario**
>
> You are a medical consultant working in a urology department in a district general hospital.
>
> A trainee approaches you stating that she has not been filling out any assessment forms since she started her training in your department. She also informs you that her colleagues have been filling and completing various forms on her behalf. When approached, she informs you that she has not been informed of the need for this process.
>
> What do you do?

## 22.1 Introduction

When presented with this scenario you will need to be able to discuss and expand on the following:

- Knowledge of trainee assessment procedures.
- Requirements for trainees' progression through their specialty training.
- Knowledge of the roles of clinical supervisors, educational supervisors and directors of regional Health Education England boards.
- The national requirements for successful completion of specialist training are outlined by the Royal Colleges and approved by the GMC/GDC.



S. Abela, *Leadership and Management in Healthcare*,
https://doi.org/10.1007/978-3-031-21025-9_22

## 22.2 Types of Trainee Assessment Tools

At the start of a training programme, each trainee should establish a learning agreement with his/her educational supervisor. Three main methods of assessment should be utilised and logged electronically on The Royal College of Surgeons of England website to allow the assessors to monitor the trainees' progression. All tools should be trainee-led and ideally supervised and graded by a consultant.

- Case-based discussion (CBD): An assessment where a trainee is given the opportunity to discuss the management of a clinical case. This is usually done during a clinical session or during an official postgraduate session.
- Direct observational procedures (DOPs): An assessment of a trainee's technical, operative and professional skills. This is usually considered from the perspective of the trainee's stage of training.
- Clinical exercises (CEXs): A clinically based exercise to monitor the trainee's skills during completion of a procedure in a clinical setting.

How is a trainee's progression assessed?

Quality assurance is usually the responsibility of a panel appointed to approve any trainee's progression.

- Review of In-Training Assessment (RITA)
- Annual Review of Competence Progression (ARCP)

The director of Health Education England (HEE) for a specific region, is usually the lead of the panel although this is not essential and an equivalent such as a deputy can be present as a replacement or completely absent if the panel does not require the director's presence.

For an Annual Review of Competence Progression (ARCP) process, at least three members from the following list have to be present:

- An external trainer.
- A Specialist accreditation committee member.
- A Royal College of Surgeons representative—this is usually a person qualified in the same speciality as the trainee.
- The Training Programme Director.
- The Educational Supervisor.
- A lay person can be appointed to chair the panel.
- An HEE support member of staff.
- University representative—this panel member is usually present for academic training posts.

The panel's objectives are as follows:

- Assess adequacy of evidence and documentation provided by the trainee.
- Analyse reports from the educational supervisors.
- Analyse the supporting documentation as set out by the specialty.
- Provide feedback.
- Assess the trainee's suitability to progress to the next stage of training or completion to be granted.

For a Review of In-Training Assessment (RITA) process, at least four members from the following list have to be present:

- Programme Director.
- A representative from the appropriate Royal College or Faculty (preferably from outside the geographical area of the training scheme).
- A representative of the consultant trainers.
- Chairman of the STC.
- Regional Specialty Advisor.
- Postgraduate Dean or his representative (usually the Associate Dean for the Specialty).
- University representative.

**The involvement of lay people in the panel**

The involvement of lay people is a requirement by the GMC. External representatives and members of the public during key stages of training are encouraged to provide:

- To ensure fairness on behalf of both the public and trainees.
- To review at least 10% of all outcomes and the evidence supporting these at random.
- Communicate with the programme director about any concerns.

All lay representatives have to undergo the recommended training including Equality and Diversity, Information Governance and Fitness to Practice. This training should be refreshed every 3 years.

Lay representatives represent the interest of the public and are responsible for raising concerns about individual trainees and the process involved.

Each HEE would have a group of trained lay persons who are actively involved in ARCP/ARCP/RITA panels, attend hospital monitoring visits, trainee interviews and are knowledgeable in trainees' requirements that ensure successful outcomes.

Our Lay representatives are encouraged to be proactive and play an active role in the above events. Following their attendance, they will provide feedback on our processes via our online report tool. The report will then be shared with the relevant HEE personnel, departments and Medical Leads to improve our policies and processes.

**Table 22.1** Key differences between ARCP and RITA processes

| | ARCP | RITA |
|---|---|---|
| Presence of trainee | Not present | Present |
| Panel's decision | Trainee informed | Decision taken in the presence of trainee |
| Evidence | Assessment of evidence | Assessment of trainee—no evidence presented |
| Outcomes | Specific to grade of trainee | Generalised and same grading are used for all types of trainees |
| Grading | Alphabetical order | Numerical order |

Lay representatives are normally assessed bi-annually using the 360-degree tool as well as self-appraisal. They are often expected to attend annual development sessions based on current hot topics.

Key differences between annual review of competence progression (ARCP) and review of the in-training assessment (RITA).

Table 22.1 lists the differences between the ARCP and RITA processes.

**Contents of a trainee's portfolio for an ARCP**

A portfolio of evidence should be compiled and presented before the panel at the ARCP meeting. A typical checklist should include the following:

A. Clinical—related documents:
   - Up-to-date Curriculum Vitae (should include new clinical and non-clinical skills acquired)
   - DOPS, CEXS and CBDs
   - 360° Multi-source feedback
   - Patient Surveys
B. Experience—related documents:
   - Patient log book
   - Teaching experience
   - Medical audits completed
   - Research projects undertaken
   - Presentations given
   - Publications in peer-reviewed journals
   - Courses attended
C. Others
   - Adverse incidents
   - Complaints

**Contents of a trainee's portfolio for a RITA**

A trainee attending a RITA process would be expected to produce the following:

- Trainers' reports and assessment forms (e.g. JCHST Yellow Form).
- The training portfolio, including CV, publications and research.

**Table 22.2** Key differences in the grading structure between the ARCP and RITA processes

| | RITA | ARCP |
|---|---|---|
| GRADE | | |
| Core information | A | No grading |
| Changes to core information | B | No grading |
| Satisfactory progress | C | 1 |
| Unsatisfactory progress | D—targeted training<br>E—Intensified training required | 2—More training needed with no additional time<br>3—More training needed with additional time<br>4—Evicted |
| Incomplete evidence | | 5 |
| Final satisfactory progress | G | 6 |
| Locum appointments for training (LATs) | | 7<br>Sub-grades:<br>7.1 Satisfactory progress<br>7.2 More competencies needed to be shown by trainee<br>7.3 Inadequate progress by trainee<br>7.4 Incomplete evidence |
| Out of programme | F | 8 |
| Fixed-term training appointments (FTTAs) | | 9<br>Sub-grades:<br>9.1 Satisfactory progress<br>9.2 More competencies needed to be shown by trainee<br>9.3 Inadequate progress by trainee<br>9.4 Incomplete evidence |

- Logbook analysis.
- Operative Competence Assessments.
- Other relevant data for the panel showing the trainee's progress.

Table 22.2 tabulates the grading differences between the ARCP and RITA processes.

## 22.3 Management of a Non-compliant Trainee

Key to managing this scenario is knowledge of the trainee's pathway, line managers involved and the educational system in your area.

Figure 22.1 illustrates the sequential management of this scenario.

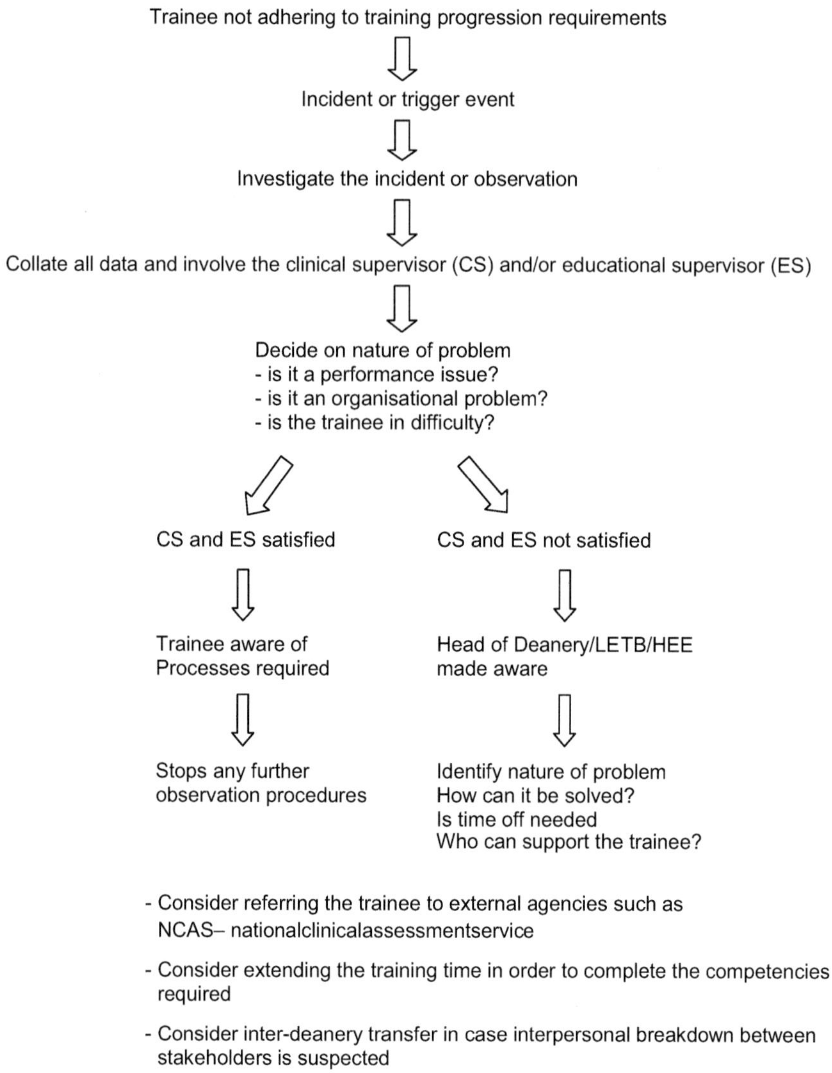


**Fig. 22.1** Algorithm for the management of a trainee in difficulty

## 22.4 Typical Trust Policies

Relevant trust policies that would offer a systematic approach and further information, respectively, to this situation are listed below in alphabetical order (the nomenclature of these policies varies between different trusts):

Policies:

- Handling concerns about a medical trainee policy.
- Managing a trainee in difficulty policy.
- Managing trainee attendance policy.
- Staff induction policy.
- Staff mandatory training and procedure policy.

# 23 Management of Recruiting New Junior Trainee

**Scenario**

You are a Consultant in dermatology, mainly based in an outpatient department in a district general hospital. You lead a small department composed of another consultant, one head nurse and two other nurses both of whom have been employed by the trust for over 10 years.

Your clinical director has suggested that the trust's management would like you to take on the trainer's role for FY1 and FY2 trainees. The department never had junior members of staff previously.

What do you do?

## 23.1 Introduction

When presented with this scenario you will need to be able to discuss and expand on the following:

- Knowledge of recruiting new members of staff.
- Knowledge of adding new trainees to the relevant regional HEE's training programme.
- Knowledge of funding streams for medical trainees.
- Ensuring quality and safety of care to patients by more junior members of staff such as FY1 and FY2 doctors.



S. Abela, *Leadership and Management in Healthcare*,
https://doi.org/10.1007/978-3-031-21025-9_23

## 23.2 Foundation Year Trainees

Following qualification as a medical doctor, the GMC grants a provisional registration on the UK's medical register. This allows a newly qualified doctor to complete a UK-approved Foundation programme.

The foundation years involve training posts for a total of 2 years following medical school and prepare trainees for eventual general practice training or specialisation. Year one of the foundation programme is known as FY1 and year two as FY2.

During the provisional registration period, a doctor can only work in FY1 approved posts and is not allowed to undertake any service posts. Exceptionally such posts could include Locum appointments of training at FY1 level.

A provisional registration can be held for a maximum of 3 years and 30 days only.

FY1 is a 1-year training post typically comprising three lots of 4 month placements.

FY2 is a further 1 year training post typically comprising four lots of 3 month placements in different specialties to broaden medical knowledge and experience.

Each Foundation Doctor must complete during each Foundation Year a minimum of:

- 6 DOPS.
- 6 Mini-CEX.
- 6 CbD.
- 2 rounds of Mini-PAT—a Multi-Source Feedback (MSF) tool which provides feedback from a range of co-workers.

The assessment tools are the same for both FY1 and FY2 years of the Foundation Programme, however, FY2 doctors should show a higher level of competence and expertise.

Successful FY1 and FY2 programmes provide eligibility for the acquisition of the Foundation Achievement of Competence Document.

Upon successful completion of F1, a certificate of experience is issued: this provides enough evidence that the requirements for full registration are met. The certificate is signed by the university, the HEE or foundation schools.

Doctors need full registration with a licence to practice to either move on to the second year of the Foundation Programme (FY2) in an approved training programme or to work in unsupervised medical practice in the NHS or UK private practice.

During the provisional registration period, a doctor can only work in FY1 approved posts and is not allowed to undertake any service posts. Exceptionally such posts could include Locum appointments of training at FY1 level.

Provisional registration can be held for a maximum of 3 years and 30 days only.

Figures 23.1 (a) and (b) illustrate the training pathway for general practitioners in the UK and Consultants, respectively, following the completion of foundation training years.

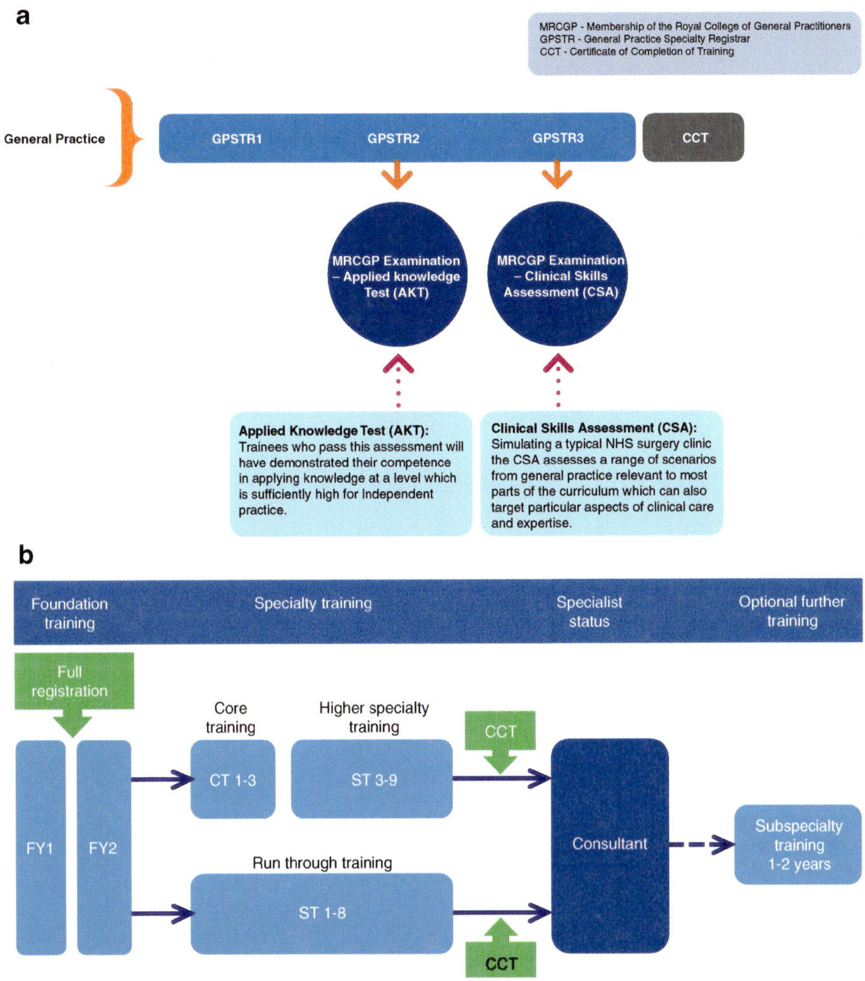


**Fig. 23.1** (**a**) Medical training pathways for general practitioners in the UK. Figure reproduced by kind permission of Health Education England. (**b**) Specialist training pathways in the UK

## 23.3 Management of Recruiting New Junior Trainees

Important considerations.

- Steps needed to set up the training posts within your directorate.
- Curriculum that needs to be delivered.
- The requirement of an attachment to a university teaching hospital and/or university.

- Establish the clinical supervisor, educational supervisor and training programme director.
- Number of supervisors that need to be involved in the programme.
- Ideal ratio of trainees to supervisors.
- Assessment of trainees' progression.
- Setting up panel and dates for ARCP meetings.
- Setting up timetable and job plans in line with the Gold Guide and with the SAC requirements.
- Physical space (office space and computer points) in the department.
- Funding stream for trainees.
- Approval by all members of staff including departmental lead, clinical director and management.
- Advertising the post on the most contemporaneous healthcare recruiting platform and on the NHS jobs website [https://www.jobs.nhs.uk].

Figure 23.2 illustrates the sequential management of this scenario.

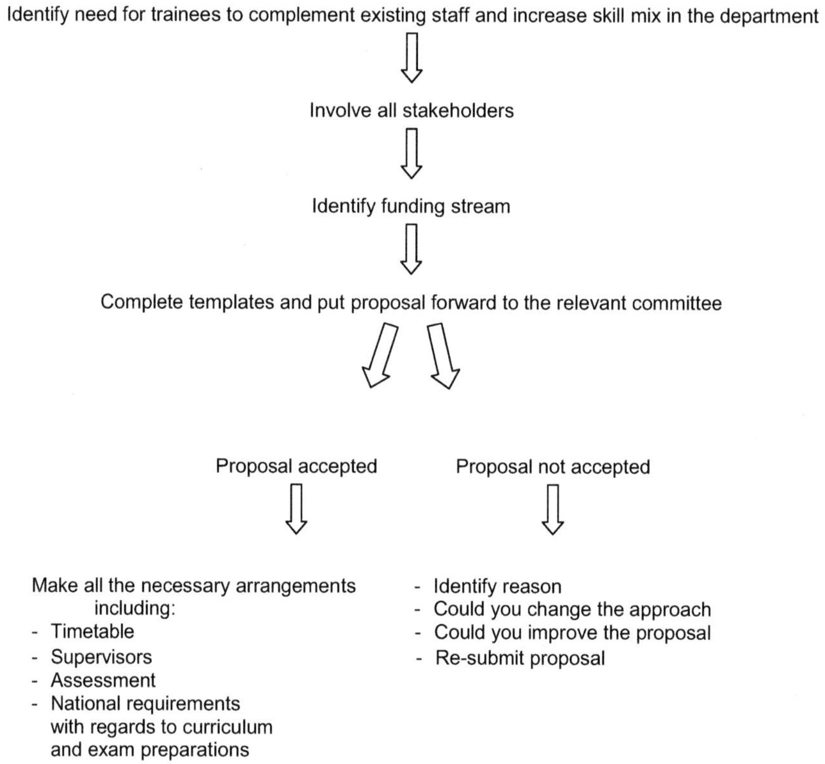


**Fig. 23.2** Flow diagram illustrating a stepwise approach to recruiting junior trainees in your department. Modified from https://www.nhsemployers.org/publications/guidance-prevention-and-management-stress-work

## 23.4 Typical Trust Policies

Relevant trust policies that would offer a systematic approach and further information, respectively, to this situation are listed below in alphabetical order (the nomenclature of these policies varies between different trusts):

Policies:

- Staff induction policy
- Staff mandatory training policy

# Management of Suspected Fraud in Your Department

# 24

> **Scenario**
> You are a consultant in Plastic Surgery specialising in breast reconstruction in a district general hospital and share an office with four other consultant colleagues. One of your colleagues is on long time sick leave and the trust has employed a new locum consultant for 4 days a week.
>
> You notice that one of his pay slips indicates the pay of a full-time equivalent.
>
> What do you do?

## 24.1 Introduction

When presented with this scenario you will need to be able to discuss and expand on the following:

- Containment of a fraud case.
- Knowledge of reporting fraud to the appropriate hospital authorities.
- Knowledge in applying the correct investigatory techniques to identify the cause.

## 24.2 Legal Framework

The management of fraud within the NHS could be simplified by using the mnemonic that could be found in the word FRAUD itself as follows:

F—Find the details of your organisation's counter fraud officer.
R—Report any concerns to your line manager.
A—Ask your local counter fraud officer to liaise with your line manager.



S. Abela, *Leadership and Management in Healthcare*,
https://doi.org/10.1007/978-3-031-21025-9_24

U—Use the organisation's policy to find out the steps on how to report a fraud suspicion.
D—Delegate investigation to the appropriate colleagues.

The question/s (Q) and answers (A) found below aim to answer any fraud-related questions that you might face in your career, in viva voces situations or in medical interviews.

Q. Which policy at your trust would address this issue?
A. Most trusts have fraud policies such as 'The Fraud Policy' which can be found on the hospital's Intranet.
Q. Which officer is likely to deal with such a situation?
A. Every trust will have an appointed officer, usually referred to as The Local Counterfraud Specialist.
Q. Which legislation would protect you if you expressed your claims?
A. The Public Interest Disclosure Act 1998 (PIDA), which gives statutory protection to individuals who report wrongdoing of a fraudulent nature.
Public Concern At Work (PCAW) is a charitable organisation which provides a whistleblowing advice line to support whistleblowers and provides up-to-date legal information.
Q. How can you classify a fraudulent activity?
A. There are four main types:

(i) Fraud: A dishonest act by an individual, or failure to report someone else for personal gain, or the committing of an offence as stipulated by the Fraud Act 2006.
(ii) Bribery: An individual imposes onto another individual or a group of people an illegal or an unethical action for personal gain. Legislation: Bribery Act 2010.
(iii) Corruption: An individual is influenced by personal gain into using his/her position to provide an advantage to someone else.
(iv) Irregularity: An act of commission or omission which might not be fraud, bribery or corruption but if left un-investigated could cause harm.

## 24.3 Management of Suspected Fraud at Work

Although every case should be treated individually due to different circumstances, every trust considers these situations as acts of gross misconduct, and a disciplinary procedure routinely ensues.

If you suspect fraudulent activity, you should repot this in accordance with your local fraud policy.

Every trust expects public employees to show; openness, probity and accountability and adherence to the Trust Standards Code of Conduct principles.

Figure 24.1 is a flow diagram illustrating sequential management of this scenario.

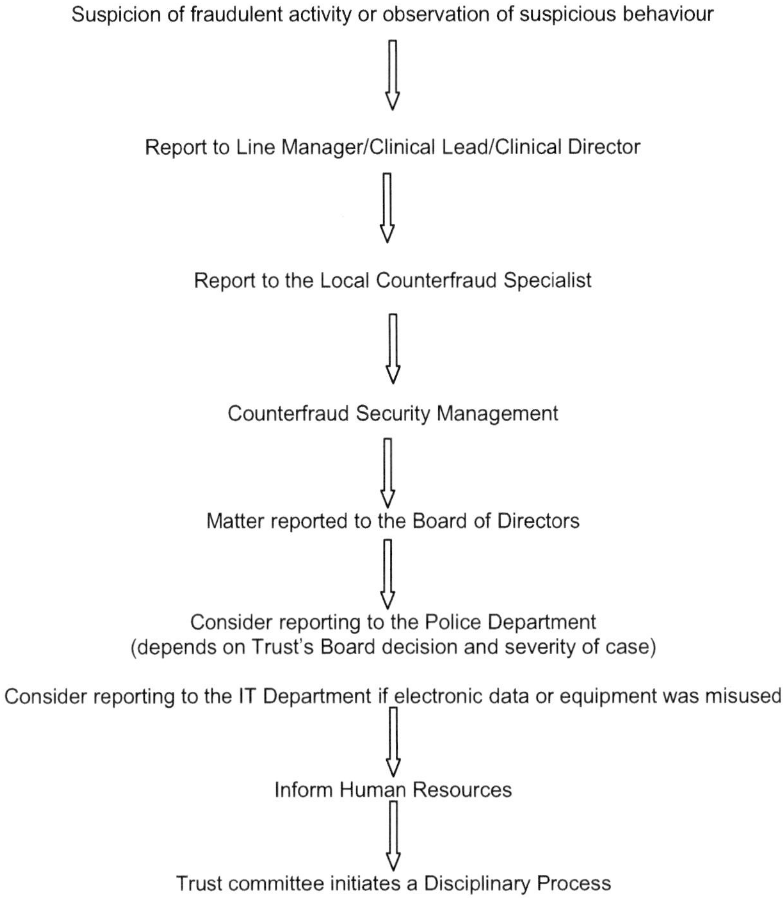


**Fig. 24.1** Management of fraudulent activity at work

## 24.4 Typical Trust Policies

Relevant trust policies that would offer a systematic approach and further information, respectively, to this situation are listed below in alphabetical order (the nomenclature of these policies varies between different trusts):

**Policies:**
- Anti-bribery policy.
- Code of conduct policy.
- Counterfraud policy.
- Disciplinary policy.
- Procurement policy.
- Whistleblowing policy.

# Management of Violence and Aggression at Work

# 25

**Scenario**

You are a specialist trainee in year 4 of your training in paediatrics and you are leading a new patient clinic for under 12-year-old patients who were referred to the hospital by their GPs due to persistent asthma.

The departmental head nurse reports to you that one of the patient's father scheduled to be seen started shouting in the waiting room and behaving violently and aggressively towards other patients sitting in the waiting room. He also starts swearing and is very impatient.

What do you do?

## 25.1 Introduction

When presented with this scenario you will need to be able to discuss and expand on the following:

- Knowledge of containing aggressive behaviour.
- Knowledge of reporting aggressive behaviour to the appropriate hospital authorities.
- Knowledge in applying the correct techniques to stop and subsequently investigate the event.



S. Abela, *Leadership and Management in Healthcare*,
https://doi.org/10.1007/978-3-031-21025-9_25

## 25.2 Legal Framework

**Which Policy at Your Trust Would Address This Issue?**
Most trusts have anti-violent and anti-abusive policies such as 'The violent and/or abusive behaviour management policy', which can be found on the hospital's intranet. The nomenclature of these policies varies between trusts.

**Which Officer Is Likely to Deal with Such a Situation?**
Every trust will have an appointed officer, usually referred to as The Local Security Management Specialist.

**Which Legislation Could You Make Use of?**
The Health and Safety Work Act 1974 provides safety regulations at work.

**What Types of Behaviour Could Be Considered Under this Policy?**
- Abuse
- Aggression
- Bullying
- Harassment
- Offensive language/gestures
- Threats
- Violence

## 25.3 Management of Violence and Aggression at Work

Trusts have a zero tolerance stance towards members of the public who demonstrate hostility, aggression or violence, or threaten staff. Trust staff can opt not to treat patients who are behaving inappropriately to staff or could be a threat to other members of the public.

In this case, the person showing aggressive behaviour is the father accompanying the patient and the treatment could carry on as scheduled unless the patient is a minor and needs the legal guardian's consent. The member of the public can be given a warning or not allowed into the premises altogether.

Figure 25.1 illustrates the management of such behaviour in the workplace.

Other actions can be considered to prevent or lessen the likelihood of a similar event happening again. The Health and Safety Executive, following a risk assessment, can propose the following:

- Environment: Improve general ambience to decrease anxiety and reduce objects that could be utilised as weapons.
- Staff training: Introduce training schemes for staff to contain aggressive episodes in an efficient and safe way.
- Staff behaviour, emotions and attitudes: Part of the staff training to improve reactions in similar scenarios.

Suspicion of aggressive or violent behaviour

↓

Take actions that can limit or decrease the act of violence. The security staff should be called who in turn would ask the aggressor to be accompanied outside the clinical area to a more private area

↓

Report to Line Manager/Clinical Lead/Clinical Director

↓

Fill in a Clinical Incident Form

↓

Report to the Local Security Management Specialist

↓

Report directly to the Health and Safety Executive Officer

↓

Matter reported to the Board of Directors

↓

Consider reporting to the Police Department
(depends on Trust's Board decision and severity of case)

↓

Inform Human Resources (if a member of staff is involved)

↓

Initiate Disciplinary Process
For staff: warning/caution/dismissal
For member of Public: issue yellow/red card and record sanction on the hospital's security system

**Fig. 25.1** Flow diagram for the management of aggressive behaviour at work

- Communicating clearly: Avoid any misleading phrases which could escalate the situation further.
- Remaining calm: Prevents additional escalation and prevents a more serious situation from occurring. This is usually part of the staff training that the trusts provide in order to manage similar situations.
- Reception areas: All patients should be attended to on arrival and any queries answered to reduce anger and aggression.
- Reducing boredom: Try to prevent long periods of waiting and inform patients of possible long waiting times beforehand.

## 25.4 Typical Trust Policies

Relevant trust policies that would offer a systematic approach and further information, respectively, to this situation are listed below in alphabetical order (the nomenclature of these policies varies between different trusts):

**Policies:**

- Dignity at work policy.
- Lone Working Policy.
- Support Staff Policy.
- Trust Security Policy.
- Violence and Aggression policy.
- Withholding Treatment Procedure Policy.
- Yellow and Red Card Policy.

# Management of Health Tourism in Your Department

# 26

**Scenario**

You are a consultant in ophthalmology at one of London's teaching hospitals.

You are leading a new patient clinic that you are assigned to once a week in the ophthalmic outpatient department. One of the patients booked on your list is a 45-year-old woman with her 12-year-old daughter who is accompanying her on that day. At the end of their appointment, following an examination, you request a 2-month follow-up appointment, at which point, the daughter admits that they will be away in Jamaica which is where they live most of the time. The mother gets angry with the daughter for stating this fact.

How would you manage this scenario if asked?

## 26.1 Introduction

When presented with this scenario you will need to be able to discuss and expand on the following:

- Knowledge of who is entitled to receive free NHS treatment.
- Management of patients not entitled to NHS treatment.
- Policies in place that deal with such situations.
- Department at the hospital which can assist you if required.

## 26.2 Legal Framework

**Which Policy at Your Trust Would Address This Issue?**

This is usually called 'The policy for overseas visitors' or 'The policy for management of patients not entitled to NHS treatment'. The title of such policies may vary between trusts.



S. Abela, *Leadership and Management in Healthcare*,
https://doi.org/10.1007/978-3-031-21025-9_26

### Which Officer Is Likely to Deal With Such a Situation?

The trust's Overseas Visitor Officer will be able to assist you to resolve such situations. Alternatively, the legal department should be able to assist any clinician with doubts over the residency of patients seeking treatment.

### What Are the Requirements Making You Eligible for NHS Treatment?

The NHS was launched by the then minister of health, Aneurin Bevan, on July 5, 1948. It has been historically based on 3 core principles:

- That it meets the needs of everyone.
- That it be free at the point of delivery.
- That it be based on clinical need, not ability to pay.

Since March 2011, the constitution of the NHS has been modified to uphold seven key principles:

1. The NHS provides a comprehensive service available to all.
2. Access to NHS services is based on clinical need, not an individual's ability to pay.
3. The NHS aspires to the highest standards of excellence and professionalism.
4. The NHS aspires to put patients at the heart of everything it does.
5. The NHS works across organisational boundaries and in partnership with other organisations in the interest of patients, local communities and the wider population.
6. The NHS is committed to providing best value for taxpayers' money and the most effective, fair and sustainable use of finite resources.
7. The NHS is accountable to the public, communities and patients that it serves.

In England, Wales and Scotland, NHS treatment is free by the respective entity, that is NHS England, NHS Wales and NHS Scotland. In Northern Ireland, Health and Social Care was created separately from the aforementioned three NHS bodies; however, it is still usually referred colloquially to as NHS Northern Ireland for simplicity purposes. Applicable fees are not dependent on the following conditions:

- Nationality.
- Payment of UK taxes.
- National Insurance contributions.
- Registration with a GP.
- Possession of an NHS number.
- Property ownership in the UK.

Since April 2015, the NHS changed the charging conditions for overseas visitors which also affected former residents of the UK. Treatment in Emergency departments and at GP surgeries remains free for all. The changes are listed below:

- Holders of a valid UK Pensioner S1 form living in an EEA country including Norway and Switzerland may be eligible to receive free healthcare in the country of residence.

- People living outside the EEA including former UK residents, have to be covered by personal health insurance and absence of this will be chargeable at 150% of the NHS national tariff for any care they receive.
  - Non-EEA nationals who apply for a visa to enter or remain in the UK for more than 6 months have to pay a surcharge.
  - Exemptions apply to UK Crown servants, British Council or Commonwealth War Graves staff and those working in UK government-funded posts overseas, residents prior to leaving the UK for government-funded posts including their spouses/civil partners and children under 18 years, armed forces members, war pensioners and armed forces compensation scheme recipients and their families, overseas residents that remain ordinarily residents in the UK despite spending time outside the UK.
- Overseas victims of violence are not charged for any condition directly caused by the act of violence experienced. The types of violence include:
  - Torture.
  - Female genital mutilation.
  - Domestic violence.
  - Sexual violence.

The exemption applies if the overseas visitor has not travelled to the UK for the purpose of seeking that treatment.

- Returning to the UK to settle will be classed as ordinarily resident, thus entitled to free NHS treatment.

**What Do Trusts Do to Identify Overseas Visitors?**
Trusts are expected to operate an efficient and effective system for the identification of overseas visitors and to ensure that any subsequent income is recovered.

All trusts should have the following:

- A proportionate procedure in place outlining the procedural steps that providers should implement to identify and collect payment from chargeable patients.
- Agreement on the information providers have to collate and how it will be shared with commissioners. UK trusts should demonstrate the capability of collating information for the commissioners to demonstrate lack of eligibility for NHS treatment.
- Agreement on how the charges are calculated depending on the care received by the non-entitled patient and how to invoice and reconcile any pending invoices.
- Undertake regular audits to ensure the commissioners that robust systems are in place to identify, collect the funds for any procedure performed and collect pending invoices.

Trusts are responsible to Identify chargeable patients:

- EEA nationals without EHIC/S2 status and submitting the information through the Department for Work and Pensions (DWP) portal.
- Non-EEA nationals, their visa status and notifying NHS Digital.

– Non-residents within the UK.
– Overseas visitors.

**What are the Basic Principles of Treating Overseas Patients?**
Where it is established that a patient is not a UK resident or has not lived here lawfully:

- The patient should be asked to complete a Pre-Attendance Form and ideally, they should be interviewed to establish their eligibility for free NHS hospital treatment.
- If the patient is from the European Economic Area or a Swiss national, visiting or temporarily living in the UK, e.g. visitors, students or temporary workers, reception staff should ask them if they have a non-UK European Health Insurance Card (EHIC) or E112 or S2 certificate. These documents allow reimbursement to the UK from the other member states.
- The person who identifies the patient as potentially liable should contact the Overseas Visitors team.
- Where it is not possible for a patient to be interviewed at the time of treatment provision this should be recorded in the health records and it is assumed that the person is liable for charges.
- Patients should always be informed about any charges.

**Should There Be any Other Arrangements?**
Every trust provides an interpreter facility which can be provided in two or three ways:

- Through an agency that allows an interpreter to accompany the patient to the hospital.
- Via a telephone conversation.
- Allowance of a family member or friend to act as an interpreter if the patient is able to fully understand what is being discussed.

It is vital for the patient to fully understand the nature of the situation or diagnosis, the options for treatment and consequences if left untreated. Validity of consent may be put into question if there is any potential lack of understanding.

**What Should You Do if You Suspect that an Overseas Patient Is Trying to Obtain Treatment They Are Not Entitled to?**
The Overseas Visitor department at your trust should be alerted immediately. If they are not available, the NHS Fraud and Corruption Reporting Line should be contacted.

## 26.3 Management of Hospital Admissions

Emergency overseas visitors are usually admitted via:

- The general practitioner.
- Self-attendance at the A&E Department.
- Transfers from other hospitals or the site of an accident.

Management of overseas patients admitted for hospital care is illustrated in Fig. 26.1.

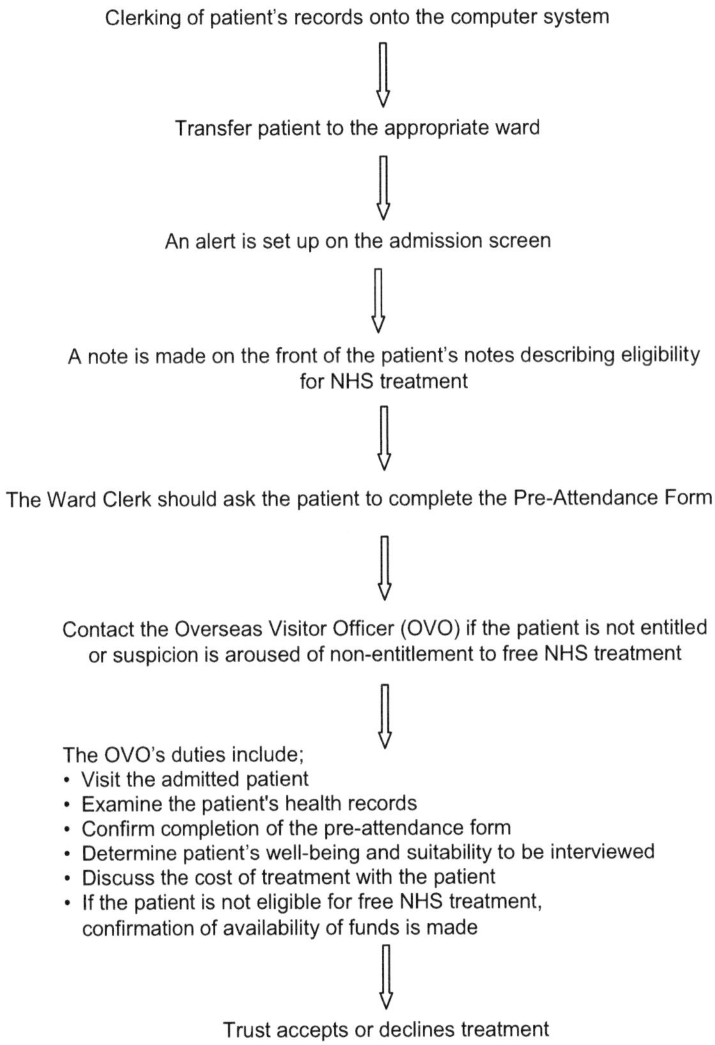


**Fig. 26.1** Stepwise procedure for the management of overseas patients admitted through A&E Department

### 26.3.1 Management of Outpatients Appointments

In this scenario, where a patient has an outpatient appointment scheduled, a few different steps should be followed (see Fig. 26.2).

The Overseas Visitor Department will:

- Request the patient reports on the day of the appointment with relevant identity documents.
- Raise a finance requisition form (some trusts refer to this form as the finance claim form) will be raised by the Overseas Visitor Officer and the payment and the full payment will be taken to the Cash Office or Billing department and the patient will be given a receipt.
- If the patient refuses to pay the cost the treating clinician would decide whether the patient has an urgent condition which requires immediate treatment.
- Some NHS services are exempt from charges and these include:
  - Accident and emergency services (unless admitted to the hospital).
  - Family planning services such as termination of a pregnancy.

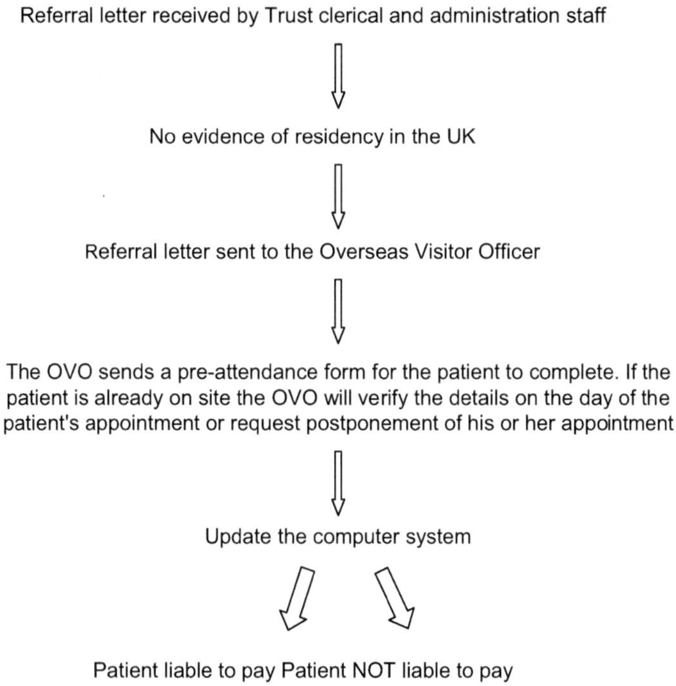


**Fig. 26.2** Stepwise procedure for the management of patients scheduled for an outpatient appointment

  - Treatment for STIs, sexually transmitted diseases.
  - Treatment for FGM, female genital mutilation, domestic or sexual violence.
- Where treatment is non-urgent, the patient should not be put on a waiting list or provided with any treatment until the patient has paid in full.

## 26.4 Patients from Countries in the European Economic Area

Any European citizen moving to the UK to work will need a visa in advance, and the employer will need to provide a sponsor licence to grant justification for the international move.

The way access to healthcare in Wales, Scotland and Northern Ireland is obtained could be different from England.

Following the accession out of the European Union, any citizen living lawfully in the UK prior to the 31st of December 2020, would not have any changes to their entitlement to NHS services.

Citizens moving to the UK after 30th of June 2021, will have to undergo immigration controls. A visa or a permit from the Home Office might be needed in order to be a lawfully abiding citizen in the UK. An immigration healthcare surcharge might be needed as part of a visa application.

Citizens exempt from this surcharge include:

- Citizens granted with IL—Indefinite Leave to remain under Part I of Appendix EU to the immigration rules, also known as 'settled status'.
- Irish citizens will not be subject to the immigration health surcharge.
- Citizens whose healthcare is paid for by an EU member state (Eligibility for full access to NHS treatment might be in full or partial with a reimbursement in line with the respective eligibility).
- Citizens based in an EU country and working in the UK.
- Family members of people of Northern Ireland.
- Children of non-UK citizens born in the UK that do not leave the country within the first three months of birth. The parents should have a valid visa of more than 6 months or have applied prior to April 2015 or have an associated healthcare surcharge paid in full or are fully exempt.

Certain charges such as prescription and/or dental charges will still apply. Family members of citizens of EU countries, Norway, Iceland, Liechtenstein or Switzerland might need to apply for a visa under the Family Rules, however, they will not be able to access free healthcare.

Students who study in the UK for less than 6 months and travel from an EU state or Norway have free access to NHS healthcare. For those travelling from Iceland, Switzerland or Liechtenstein may not be eligible for free NHS access, chargeable at 150% of the NHS rate.

Students staying in the UK for longer than 6 months will need to go through a visa process with any associated healthcare surcharges. The following conditions might make a student eligible for a partial or full reimbursement:

- Full-time UK higher education.
- Visa status started on or after the first of January 2021.
- Possession of a valid EHIC issued in an EU country.
- Not a registered worker or employee in the UK.

EU citizens can access NHS care, using four main documents:

- European Health Insurance Card (EHIC).
- Provisional Replacement Certificate (PRC)—in the absence of an EHIC.
- S1 form.
- S2 form.

**European Health Insurance Card (EHIC)**
European Health Insurance Cards (EHICs) are used by EU visitors and students travelling to the UK. The UK will in turn claim for any healthcare-related costs from the respective country. This applies to procedures that are deemed an emergency and cannot be delayed till the patient returns to his or her's country of origin.

**Provisional Replacement Certificate (PRC)—Patients without an EHIC**
A Provisional Replacement Certificate (PRC) is issued by the hospital where the patient is receiving treatment due to the non-availability of an EHIC.

**S1 Form**
S1 forms are healthcare certificates issued to citizens who live in one EU country but have their healthcare costs covered by another EU country.

People entitled to S1 forms include:

- State pensioners.
- Citizens in receipt of certain benefits, for example survivors' benefits and certain disability benefits.
- Citizens who have been posted to work in another country (full-time residence for more than two years).
- Frontier workers, commuting across borders for work purposes.
- Family members of citizens entitled to the S1 form.

**S2 Form**

S2 forms are issued to citizens covered by a reciprocal healthcare arrangement who choose to have their healthcare in an EU country of their choice.

## 26.5 Typical Trust Policies and Relevant Documents

Relevant trust policies that would offer a systematic approach and further information, respectively, to this situation are listed below in alphabetical order (the nomenclature of these policies varies between different trusts):

**Policies:**

- Management of patients not eligible for NHS treatment policy.
- Overseas visitor policy.

**Relevant Documents:**

- Department of Health and Social Care (2012) Guidance on implementing the overseas visitor charging regulations, Guidance, October 2012.
  [https://assets.publishing.service.gov.uk/government/uploads/system/uploads/attachment_data/file/213015/GUIDANCE-October-2012-FINAL.pdf—accessed January 2020]
- NHS England (2015) The Handbook to The NHS Constitution; a handbook, July 2015.
- [https://assets.publishing.service.gov.uk/government/uploads/system/uploads/attachment_data/file/480482/NHS_Constitution_WEB.pdf—accessed January 2020]
- NHS England (2015) Improving Systems for Cost Recovery for Overseas Visitors; guidance March 2015.
- [https://www.england.nhs.uk/wp-content/uploads/2018/02/improving-systems-guidance-chargeable-overseas-visitor.pdf—accessed January 2020].

# Management of Colleagues Affected by Stress at Work

# 27

> **Scenario**
>
> You are a consultant in an orthopaedic department in a district general hospital. The department has got five consultants in orthopaedics in total.
>
> You had a request to assist a colleague who is finding managing a clinic a 'bit' difficult. The nurse leading the clinic asks you to help out because the patients have been waiting too long for their consultations. Your colleague is also showing a change in mood and is becoming easily irritated. You have also noticed that he booked three new patients in the wrong clinic.
>
> What should you do?

## 27.1 Introduction

When presented with this scenario you will need to be able to discuss and expand on the following:

- Knowledge of how to support colleagues and be part of a team.
- Identification of stress at work.
- Policies in place that deal with such situations.
- Which department at the hospital can assist you if required.

Stress is the consequence of a 'stressor' which is a stimulus that leads to stress. It is very common in the workplace and affects approximately 20% of the workforce or one in five adults in the UK at any one time, whilst in general around one in two people will experience stress in their lifetime.



S. Abela, *Leadership and Management in Healthcare*,
https://doi.org/10.1007/978-3-031-21025-9_27

It is estimated that three-quarters of visits to the GP in the UK are stress related.

Possible causes are varied and differ between individuals. Below is a list of possible causes:

- Life events—The most traumatic life events are marital separation, imprisonment and death of a close family member in decreasing order. Other stressful life events include personal injury, illness, dismissal from work and retirement.
- Negative outlook—A negative work experience can impose a long-term negative outlook which has long-lasting effects on an individual's desire to progress and change jobs.
- Anger—An individual has to manage feelings of anger.
- Personality—People with different personalities react differently to stress.

## 27.2 Stress at Work

The Health and Safety Executive defines stress as 'the adverse reaction people have to excessive pressure or other types of demand placed on them'.

**Trust Policies Relevant to this Scenario**

Trust policies such as the 'Stress at work policy' should be found on the trust intranet. Other relevant policies, guidelines and supporting documents can also be found such as:

- Risk assessment form and procedure.
- Serious untoward incidents policy.
- Violence and abusive behaviour management policy.
- Bullying and harassment policy.
- Stress at work policy.
- Complaints handling policy.

**What is the Immediate Support for Staff Experiencing Stress at Work?**

Staff experiencing health symptoms related to workplace stress can go unnoticed, often due to workplace demands and the experience could be ongoing for some time before the affected member of staff seeks support.

**What is the Immediate Support for Staff Experiencing Stress at Work?**

Any affected members of staff should have access to immediate support from their employer. This is readily available via the following channels:

- Through their line manager.
- Through their divisional manager.

- Via the employers' workplace Health and Wellbeing Department (this department's nomenclature varies between trusts; other names could include Occupational Health and Wellbeing Department, Staff Health and Wellbeing Department, The Occupational Health Department amongst others).
- Via the commissioned counselling advisors offered by your employer. As an example, if you are a doctor working for a trust based in the North East of the United Kingdom, free support sessions would be provided by Insight Healthcare.

**Insight Healthcare**

Url: https://www.insighthealthcare.org

Insight Healthcare is a non-profit organisation that offers free talking therapy sessions to NHS employees in several locations in the United Kingdom. Insight Healthcare forms part of the Concern Group which seeks to improve the health and mental well-being of individuals. The assistance programme available at your trust can be found on the hospital's intranet by identifying the relevant policy or section.

Staff can also self-refer confidentially by organising an appointment with their workplace Health and Well-being, department directly.

**Which Officer is Likely to Deal with Such a Situation?**

An occupational health officer, together with the employee's general practitioner and his or her line manager can offer help and support. Human resources or medical staffing would also get involved if time off work is required.

The Lead Health and Safety Advisor together with the trust's Health and Safety Committee could be involved if the situation escalates and patients' safety is at risk.

Referral of the affected individual to the Occupational Health department is usually done through the line manager, or occasionally through self-referral, confidentially. The employee has the right to withhold any medical or other confidential information from the line manager.

**Importance of Identifying Stress at Work**

Stress can lead to:

- Inefficiency at work (taking much longer to finish a task).
- Unpleasant work environment.
- Longer and more frequent absenteeism.
- Underperformance with multiple mistakes, oversights and omissions of tasks.

Table 27.1 tabulates the identifying signals of stress at work.

**Table 27.1** Identifying signals of stress at work

**Changes and Signs of Stress at Work**

| | |
|---|---|
| **Behavioural Changes** | - New Habits/Vices such as; increased drinking and/or smoking<br>- Increasingly irritable<br>- Avoiding People and decreasing social contact with other members of staff<br>- Multiple episodes of absenteeism<br>- Change in appetite |
| **Mental Signs** | - Multiple errors<br>- Indecisiveness<br>- Memory lapses<br>- Shifting responsibilities<br>- Worrying mistakes<br>- No interest at work<br>- No commitment<br>- Late arrival and early departure<br>- Lack of teamwork |
| **Physical Changes** | - lack of concentration<br>- signs of fatigue<br>- feeling exhausted<br>- frequent feeling of dizziness<br>- indigestion<br>- breathlessness |
| **Emotional Signs** | - crying<br>- bad temper<br>- sulking<br>- no sense of humour<br>- dramatisation of facts |

**Implementing the Department's Policy**

It is the responsibility of line managers to ensure adherence to, and implementation of the policy to minimise 'stressors' at work.

Staff—Discuss and disclose concerns about any stress-causing factors. Obtain the appropriate training and be knowledgeable in filling the Stress Identification Form (the name of this form might vary between trusts). All staff should be aware of how to obtain further advice and guidance from the Occupational Health department and/or trade union if necessary.

**Line Managers** The line manager of the department or ward has to implement the policy and complete the annual department inspection checklist, which includes a review of the department's workplace stress risk assessment.

Line managers should also be able to complete an individual stress risk assessment form. This is normally done following a self-referring member of staff within the department, following a GP report, or advice from the Occupational Health department.

**Divisional Managers** Divisional managers should keep abreast of the trust policies and any updates and actions if needed.

**Occupational Health Department (OH)** Occupational Health is trained to provide support, advice and guidance to the member of staff undergoing a stressful period. The department will also provide support and guidance to the staff's line manager and offer independent counselling advice to the staff member.

Following a 'rehabilitation' period, the department produces a report to the Health and Safety Committee.

**Chief Executive (CE)** The CE is ultimately responsible for ensuring safe and stress-free working environment.

Sequential Management of an individual experiencing stress:

1. Identify the 'stressor'.
2. The affected individual self-refers by submitting a stress identification form, sickness absence is reported by his or her general practitioner or following the advice from OH.
3. The line manager completes a stress risk assessment form and identifies the potential risk of other individuals being affected. The line manager takes appropriate action to relieve the 'stressor' and if this is not possible support from more senior managers should be sought.
4. Local OH involvement.
5. Referral to an independent counselling provider.

**Management Standards for Work-Related Stress**

The Management Standards issued by the Health and Safety Executive (HSE) are the standards adopted by trusts to assist in the reduction and management of work-related stress.

HSE is an Executive non-department public body (NDPB) of the Department for Work and Pensions with its main being that of reducing work-related injury which results in absence from work.

The Management Standards cover six key areas of work design that, if not properly managed, could lead to work-related stress.

The primary sources of stress at work are listed below:

- Demands: No say or no flexibility on issues such as workload, work patterns and the work environment.
- Control: Employees' opinions are not valued and conditions requested by the members of staff are not met by their line managers.
- Support: No recognition or support by the organisation, line management and colleagues.
- Relationships: No structure or framework in place to avoid conflicts and quick resolution pathways if this occurs.
- Role: No clear role within the organisation hierarchy.
- Change: The absence of a framework to disseminate positive work changes.

The Management Standards offer:

- Demonstration of good practice through a step-by-step risk assessment approach.
- Assessment of the current situation.
- Promotion of active discussion and involvement of all employees.
- Simplified risk assessment for work-related stress by:
  - Identifying the main risk factors for work-related stress.
  - Helping employers focus on the underlying causes and their prevention.
  - Providing a yardstick by which organisations can gauge their performance in tackling the key causes of stress.

## 27.3 Stepwise Approach Following Identification of Stress at Work

A stepwise approach to manage stress at work is illustrated in Fig. 27.1.

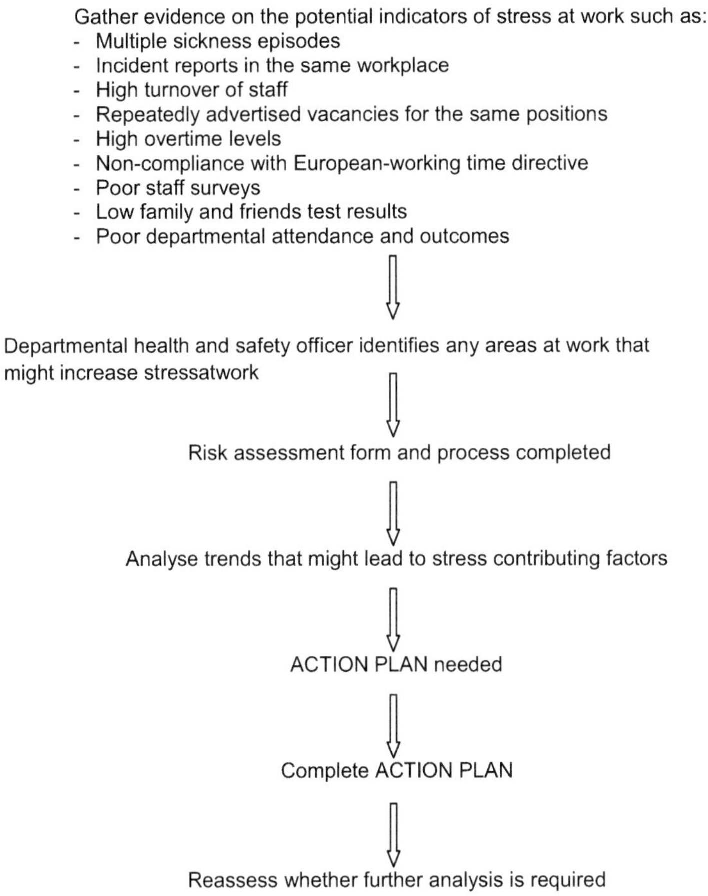


**Fig. 27.1** Management of a stressed colleague within your department. Modified from https://www.nhsemployers.org/publications/guidance-prevention-and-management-stress-work

## 27.4 Legislations and Typical Trust Policies

**Legislations:**

– Health and Safety at Work Act 1974 available online via: http://www.legislation.gov.uk/ukpga/1974/37/pdfs/ukpga_19740037_en.pdf, accessed January 2020
– HSE Health and Safety at Work Regulations 1999 available online via: http://www.legislation.gov.uk/uksi/1999/3242/pdfs/uksi_19993242_en.pdf, accessed January 2020.

Relevant trust policies that would offer a systematic approach and further information, respectively, to this situation are listed below in alphabetical order (the nomenclature of these policies varies between different trusts):

**Policies:**
- Bullying and harassment policy.
- Complaints handling policy.
- Health and Safety at Work Regulations.
- Serious untoward incidents policy.
- Stress at work policy.
- Violence and abusive behaviour management policy.

## 27.5 Sources of Further Information

- Department for Work and Pensions (2016) Framework document between The Health and Safety Executive and The Department for Work and Pensions, January 2016. [http://data.parliament.uk/DepositedPapers/Files/DEP2016-0071/DWP_HSE_FRAMEWORK_DOCUMENT_2016.pdf, accessed August 2018].
- HSE website: www.hse.gov.uk/stress

# Management of Inappropriate Use of Social Media

# 28

**Scenario**

You are the clinical lead.

You are called by the clinical director requesting some information about a photograph that has appeared on a social media website. This photograph shows a group of your nurses partying and displaying signs of inappropriate behaviour with the hospital's uniform clearly on display.

How would you manage such a situation?

## 28.1 Introduction

When presented with this scenario you will need to be able to discuss and expand on the following:

- Knowledge of appropriate behaviour when representing the trust.
- Management of information disseminated via social media.
- Policies in place that deal with such situations.
- Which department at the hospital can assist you if required.



S. Abela, *Leadership and Management in Healthcare*,
https://doi.org/10.1007/978-3-031-21025-9_28

## 28.2 Use of Social Media at Work

The key aspect with regards to the use of social media revolves around the forbidden sharing of patients' confidential information or inappropriate behaviour which is not in line with the employing organisations values.

The medical, dental, nursing and the health and care professions regulations have guidance on the use of social media. Below are online links to each of the regulator's guidances:

General Medical Council (2013) Doctor's use of social media. Url: https://www.gmc-uk.org/-/media/documents/gmc-guidance-for-doctors%2D%2D-doctors-use-of-social-media_pdf-58833100.pdf - accessed September 2022.

General Dental Council (2016) Guidance on using social media. Url: https://www.gdc-uk.org/docs/default-source/guidance-documents/guidance-on-using-social-media.pdf?sfvrsn=de158345_2 - accessed September 2022.

Nursing and Midwifery Council (2013) Guidance on using social media responsibly. Url: https://www.nmc.org.uk/globalassets/sitedocuments/nmc-publications/social-media-guidance.pdf - accessed September 2022.

Health and Care Professions Council (2017) Guidance on social media. Url: https://www.hcpc-uk.org/globalassets/resources/guidance/guidance-on-social-media.pdf - accessed September 2022.

**Which Policy at Your Trust Would Address This Issue?**

The 'Social media policy' would address this scenario. However, other policies such as 'Being open', the 'Speak up policy' or 'Whistleblowing policy' could also be relevant. The 'Conduct and capability policy' and 'The cyber code of conduct' are other relevant policies that could apply.

**Social Media Sites**

Inappropriate behaviour on social media arises when staff utilise these websites/apps to disrespect the values and policies of the trust. The employee's contract is likely to contain a section highlighting the careful use of social media out of work hours and out of the hospital premises.

**Social Media Trust policy's Principle at your Trust**
The main scope of your trusts' social media policy is to advice against the use of social media that can portray staff behaving in ways that could potentially compromise the trust's reputation.

**The Trust's Expectations of its Employees**
When identifiable as a trust staff member, employees should:

- Not reveal confidential information about any patient, staff member or information belonging to the trust.
- Not engage in activities on the Internet which might bring the trust into disrepute.
- Not transfer identifiable personal information that can result in identity transfer.
- Not use the Internet to disclose personal information about other colleagues.
- Not post defamatory, derogatory or offensive comments on the Internet about other employees of the trust.
- In the case of senior members of staff, set an example to younger members of the team.
- Only use Internet sites and social media to socialise respectfully and in a constructive manner.

**Relevant Definitions**
Derogatory—Tending to detract from, involving impairment, disparagement or discredit.

Defamatory—Harmful and often untrue; tending to discredit or malign.

Disrepute—Ill repute, discredit.

Discredit—Refuse to believe, bring disbelief or disrepute upon.

## 28.3 Stepwise Management Following Incident

Figure 28.1 illustrates the sequential management of colleagues misusing social medial platforms.

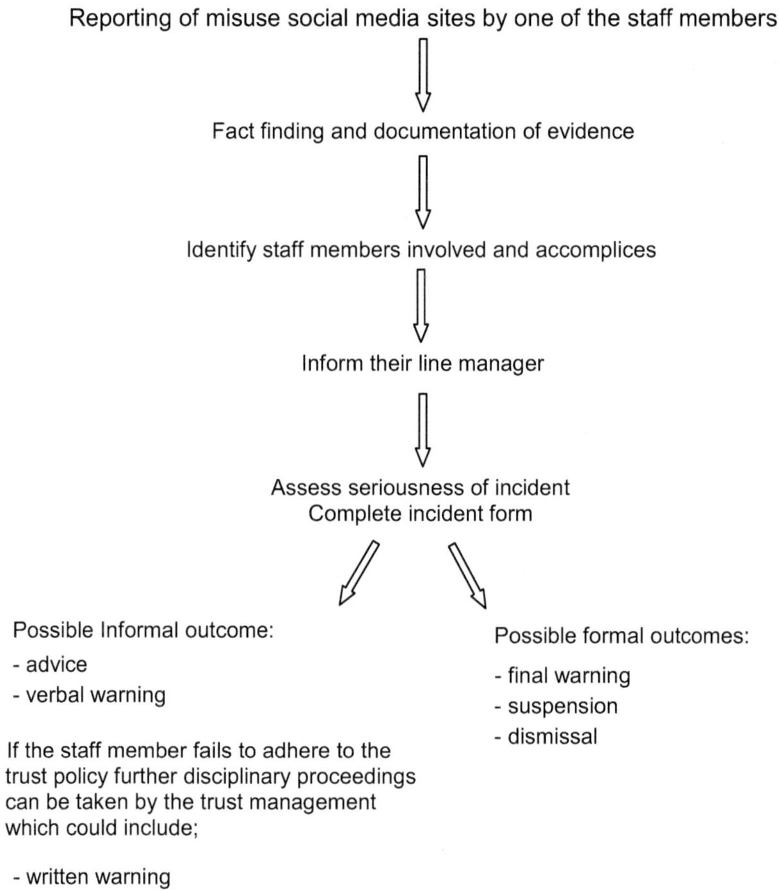


**Fig. 28.1** Flow diagram illustrating the steps needed to be taken in case of social media misuse

## 28.4 Legislations and Typical Trust Policies

**Legislations:**

- Data Protection Act 1998
- Defamation Act 1996
- Equality Act 2010
- Human Rights Act 1998

Relevant trust policies that would offer a systematic approach and further information, respectively, to this situation are listed below in alphabetical order (the nomenclature of these policies varies between different trusts):

**Policies:**

- Being open.
- Conduct and capability policy.
- Email use policy.
- Internet use policy.
- Social media policy The cyber code of conduct.
- Speak up policy.
- Whistleblowing policy.

# Appendix 1

List of commonly asked Acts and Legislations

**A**
Access to Health Records Act 1990
Url: https://www.legislation.gov.uk/ukpga/1990/23/pdfs/ukpga_19900023_en.pdf - Accessed January 2020
Access to Medical Reports Acts 1988
Url: https://www.legislation.gov.uk/ukpga/1988/28/pdfs/ukpga_19880028_en.pdf - Accessed January 2020
**C**
Children Act 2004
Url: https://www.legislation.gov.uk/ukpga/2004/31/pdfs/ukpga_20040031_en.pdf - Accessed January 2020
Computer Misuse Act 1990
Url: https://www.legislation.gov.uk/ukpga/1990/18/pdfs/ukpga_19900018_en.pdf - Accessed January 2020
Control of Misleading Advertising Act 1998
Url: http://www.legislation.gov.uk/uksi/1988/915/made?view=plain - Accessed January 2020
Criminal Justice Act 2003
Url: https://www.legislation.gov.uk/ukpga/2003/44/pdfs/ukpga_20030044_en.pdf - Accessed January 2020
**D**
Data Protection Act 1998
Url: https://www.legislation.gov.uk/ukpga/1998/29/pdfs/ukpga_19980029_en.pdf - Accessed August 2018
Data Protection Act 2018
Url: http://www.legislation.gov.uk/ukpga/2018/12/pdfs/ukpga_20180012_en.pdf - Accessed January 2020
Disability Discrimination Act 1995
Url: http://www.legislation.gov.uk/ukpga/1995/50/pdfs/ukpga_19950050_en.pdf - Accessed January 2020
**E**
Employment Equality Regulations 2003
Url: http://www.legislation.gov.uk/uksi/2003/1660/pdfs/uksi_20031660_en.pdf - Accessed January 2020
Equalities Act 2010
Url: https://www.legislation.gov.uk/ukpga/2010/15/pdfs/ukpga_20100015_en.pdf - Accessed January 2020



S. Abela, *Leadership and Management in Healthcare*,
https://doi.org/10.1007/978-3-031-21025-9

**F**

Freedom of Information Act 2000

Url: https://www.legislation.gov.uk/ukpga/2000/36/pdfs/ukpga_20000036_en.pdf - Accessed January 2020

**H**

Health Care and Associated Professions (Indemnity Arrangements) Order 2014

Url: http://www.legislation.gov.uk/uksi/2014/1887/pdfs/uksi_20141887_en.pdf - Accessed January 2020

Health and Safety Act 1974

Url: https://www.legislation.gov.uk/ukpga/1974/37/pdfs/ukpga_19740037_en.pdf - Accessed January 2020

Human Rights act 2000

Url: https://www.legislation.gov.uk/ukpga/1998/42/pdfs/ukpga_19980042_en.pdf - Accessed January 2020

**P**

Privacy and Electronic Communications Regulations 2003

Url: http://www.legislation.gov.uk/uksi/2003/2426/pdfs/uksi_20032426_en.pdf - Accessed January 2020

Protection from Harassment Act 1997

Url: https://www.legislation.gov.uk/ukpga/1997/40/pdfs/ukpga_19970040_en.pdf - Accessed January 2020

Public Interest Disclosure Act 1998

Url: https://www.legislation.gov.uk/ukpga/1998/23/pdfs/ukpga_19980023_en.pdf - Accessed January 2020

Public Records Act 1998

Url: http://www.legislation.gov.uk/ukpga/1958/51/pdfs/ukpga_19580051_en.pdf - Accessed January 2020

**R**

Race Relations Act 1995

Url: http://www.legislation.gov.uk/ukpga/1976/74/pdfs/ukpga_19760074_en.pdf - Accessed January 2020

Rehabilitation of Offenders Act 1974

Url: https://www.legislation.gov.uk/ukpga/1974/53/pdfs/ukpga_19740053_en.pdf - Accessed January 2020

**S**

Sex Discrimination Act 1975

Url: https://www.legislation.gov.uk/ukpga/1975/65/pdfs/ukpga_19750065_en.pdf - Accessed January 2020

Sexual Offences Act 2003

Url: http://www.legislation.gov.uk/ukpga/2003/42/pdfs/ukpga_20030042_en.pdf - January 2020

**T**

The Corporate Manslaughter and Corporate Homicide Act 2007

Url: http://www.legislation.gov.uk/ukpga/2007/19/pdfs/ukpga_20070019_en.pdf - Accessed January 2020

The Dentists Act 1984

Url: http://www.legislation.gov.uk/ukpga/1984/24/pdfs/ukpga_19840024_en.pdf - Accessed January 2020

The Medical Act 1983

Url: http://www.legislation.gov.uk/ukpga/1983/54/pdfs/ukpga_19830054_en.pdf - Accessed January 2020

The Regulations of Investigatory Powers Act 2000

Url: https://www.legislation.gov.uk/ukpga/2000/23/pdfs/ukpga_20000023_en.pdf - Accessed January 2020

# Appendix 2

Listed in alphabetical order, are typical trust policies commonly asked by UK trusts. Please note that the nomenclature used by different trusts may vary. It is very important that the reader is aware of the names and summary of contents of these policies as they form the basis of interview questions, management principles, management exam questions and day-to-day management know-how for every medical doctor and dental surgeon based in a hospital setting.

| |
|---|
| **A** |
| Adoption leave policy |
| Annual leave policy |
| Anti-bribery policy |
| **B** |
| Being open policy |
| **C** |
| Capability policy |
| Capital Expenditure policy |
| Career break policy |
| Children with multiple failed to attend policy |
| Claims management policy |
| Clinical audit policy |
| Code of business conduct policy |
| Complaints procedure policy |
| Consent procedure policy |
| Control of substances hazardous to health procedure policy |
| Criminal check records policy |
| Cyber code of conduct policy |
| Cytotoxic spillage procedure policy |
| **D** |
| Data protection policy |
| Data quality policy |
| Digital images and confidential data handling policy |
| Dignity at work policy |
| Disciplinary procedure policy |
| **F** |
| Fraud and corruption policy |


S. Abela, *Leadership and Management in Healthcare*,
https://doi.org/10.1007/978-3-031-21025-9

**G**
Grievance procedure policy
**I**
Investigating incidents, complaints and claims reporting procedure policy
**J**
Job sharing policy
**L**
Leavers procedure policy
**M**
Major incident procedure
Maternity leave policy
**N**
New therapy and interventions procedure
**O**
Overseas visitors policy
**P**
Paternity leave policy
Patient access policy
Policy for the identification and assessment, recording and management of risks on the Risk Register
Prevention and management of needlestick and sharps injuries
Probationary period policy
Professional registration policy
**R**
Reporting and management of incidents, near misses and serious incidents policy
Reporting of injuries, diseases and dangerous occurrences policy
Retirement procedure policy
**S**
Safeguarding children policy
Safeguarding vulnerable adults policy
Slips, trips and falls policy
Social media policy
Speak-out policy (whistleblowing policy)
Staff induction policy
Staff mandatory training policy
Stress at work policy
Study leave policy
Substance misuse policy
**U**
Unexplained injuries in children policy
Uniform policy
**V**
Violent and aggressive behaviour policy
Voluntary Severance scheme policy
**W**
Work experience policy

# Appendix 3

Measurement of the Risk Score

The appendix below has been reproduced, courtesy of NHS England from the document entitled 'A Risk Matrix for Risk Managers' by the National Patient Safety Agency, 2008, under the Open Government Licence.

| | Consequence score (severity levels) and examples of descriptors | | | | |
|---|---|---|---|---|---|
| | 1 | 2 | 3 | 4 | 5 |
| **Domains** | **Negligible** | **Minor** | **Moderate** | **Major** | **Catastrophic** |
| **Impact on the safety of patients, staff or public (physical/psychological harm)** | Minimal injury requiring no/minimal intervention or treatment<br>No time off work required | Minor injury or illness requiring minor intervention<br>Requiring time off work for <3 days<br>Increase is length of hospital stay by 1–3 days | Moderate injury requiring professional intervention<br>Requiring time off work for 4-14 days<br>Increase in length of hospital stay by 4-15 days<br>RIDDOR/agency reportable incident<br>An event which impacts on a small number of patients | Major injury leading to long-term incapacity/disability<br>Requiring time off work for >14days<br>Increase in length of hospital stay by>15 days<br>Mismanagement of patient care with long-term effects | Incident leading to death<br>Multiple permanent injuries or irreversible health effects<br>An event which impacts on a large number of patients |
| **Quality/complaints/audit** | Peripheral element of treatment or service sub-optimal<br>Informal complaint/inquiry | Ovetall treatment or service sub-optimal<br>Formal complaint (stage 1)<br>Local resolution<br>Single failure to meet internal standards<br>Minor implications for patient safety if unresolved<br>Reduced performance rating if unresolved | Treatment or service has significantly reduced effectiveness<br>Formal complaint (stage 2)<br>Local resolution (with potential to go to independent review)<br>Repeated failure to meet internal standards<br>Major patient safety implications if findings are not acted on | Non-compliance with national standards with significant risk to patients if unresolved<br>Multiple complaints/independent review<br>Low performance rating<br>Critical report | Incident leading to totally unacceptable level or quality of treatment/service<br>Gross failure of patient safety if findings not acted on<br>Inquest/ombudsman inquiry<br>Gross failure to meet national standards |



S. Abela, *Leadership and Management in Healthcare*,
https://doi.org/10.1007/978-3-031-21025-9

## Index

| | | | | | |
|---|---|---|---|---|---|
| **Human resources/ Organisational development/ staffing/competence** | Short-term low staffing level that temporarily reduces service quality (<1 day) | Low staffing level that redces service quality | Late delivery of key objective/ service due to lack of staff<br>Unsafe staffing level or competence (>1day)<br>Low staff morale<br>Poor staff attendance for mandatory/key training | Uncertain delivery of key objective/service due to lack of staff<br>Unsafe staffing level or competence (>5 days)<br>Loss of key staff<br>Very low staff morale<br>No staff attendance for mandatory/key training | Non-delivery of key objective/service due to lack of staff<br>Ongoing unsafe staffing levels or competence<br>Loss of several key staff<br>No staff attending mandatory training/key training on an ongoing basis |
| **Statutory duty/ inspections** | No or minimal impact or breed, of guidance/ statutory duty | Breach of statutory legislation<br>Reduced performance rating if unresolved | Single breech in statutory duty<br>Challenging external recommendations/ improvement notice | Enforcement action<br>Multiple breeches in statutory duty<br>Improvement notices<br>Low performance rating<br>Critical report | Multiple breeches in statutory duty<br>Prosecution<br>Complete systems change required<br>Zero performance rating<br>Severely critical report |
| **Finance including claims** | Small loss<br>Risk of claim remote | Loss of 0.1–0.25 per cent of budget<br>Claim less than £10,000 | Loss of 0.25–0.5 per cent of budget<br>Claim(s) between £10,000 and £100,000 | Uncertain delivery of key objective/Loss of 0.5–1.0 per cent of budget<br>Claim(s) between £100,000 and £1 million<br>Purchasers failing to pay on time | Non-delivery of key objective/loss of > 1 per cent of budget<br>Failure to meet specification/ slippage<br>Loss of contract/ payment by results<br>Claim(s) >£1 million |
| **Service/business interruption**<br>**Environmental Impact** | Loss/interruption of > 1 hour<br>Minimal or no impact on the environment | Loss/interruption of >8 hours<br>Minor impact on environment | Loss/interruption of >1 day<br>Moderate impact on environment | Loss/interruption of >1 week<br>Major impact on environment | Permanent loss of service or facility<br>Catastrophic impact on environment |

# The Glossary

| | |
|---|---|
| Arm's-length body | A non-departmental public body independent of government |
| CCGs (Clinical Commissioning Groups) | Commission health services at a local level |
| Clinical Senates | Provide independent strategic and clinical advice for CCGs |
| Commissioning | Process by which services are planned and provided effectively to meet the specific needs of the local population |
| CQC (Care Quality Commission) | The independent regulator of health and social care in England |
| CQUIN (Commissioning for Quality and Innovation) | A financial incentive to improve quality of services and achieve better outcomes |
| CSU (Commissioning Support Unit) | Provide support to CCGs, NHS England, acute trusts and government |
| DH (Department of Health) | Branch of UK government responsible for health and social care policy and legislation |
| FT (Foundation Trust) | Delivers care to the population and has autonomy in the day-to-day running of operations |
| Healthwatch | Independent consumer champion; its role is to represent the views of patients |
| HEE (Health Education England) | A special health authority providing leadership for new education and training systems for healthcare professionals |
| HWB (Health and Wellbeing Board) | A forum which brings key leaders across the healthcare system together to improve health and address inequalities in a local population |
| ICS (Integrated Care Systems) | A partnership of organisations responsible for delivery care to their respective geographical area in which they are based |
| LETB (Local Education and Training Board) | Responsible for training and education of clinical and non-clinical NHS staff in their area |
| Monitor | NHS regulator that supports organisations which purchase and provide health care to make decisions in the best interest of patients Monitor became part of NHS Improvement in April 2016 |
| NHS England | A non-departmental public body of the DH; oversees the budget, planning, delivery and day-to-day operations of the NHS in England |
| NHSI (NHS Improvement) | Works with the Department of Health and Social Care to oversee NHS Foundation trusts and ensure optimal healthcare delivery |



S. Abela, *Leadership and Management in Healthcare*,
https://doi.org/10.1007/978-3-031-21025-9

| | |
|---|---|
| NHS TDA (Trust Development Authority) | Responsible for providing leadership and support to non-foundation trusts |
| NICE (National Institute for Health and Care Excellence) | Provides national guidance and advice to improve health and social care; provides a database to encourage the use of evidence-based medicine |
| PHE (Public Health England) | An executive agency of the DH that aims to protect and improve the nation's health and address inequalities |
| PPA (Practitioner Performance Advice) | Provide impartial advice to healthcare bodies and health care professionals including doctors, dentists and pharmacists to resolve safety concerns |

Printed by Printforce, the Netherlands